Student Solutions Manual

for use with

A Guide to
Good Reasoning

David C. Wilson
UCLA

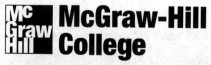

McGraw-Hill College

Boston   Burr Ridge, IL   Dubuque, IA   Madison, WI
New York   San Francisco   St. Louis
Bangkok   Bogotá   Caracas   Lisbon   London   Madrid   Mexico City
Milan   New Delhi   Seoul   Singapore   Sydney   Taipei   Toronto

McGraw-Hill College

A Division of The McGraw·Hill Companies

Student Solutions Manual for use with
A GUIDE TO GOOD REASONING

1 2 3 4 5 6 7 8 9 0 EDW/EDW 9 3 2 1 0 9 8

ISBN 0-07-233244-1

http://www.mhhe.com

TABLE OF CONTENTS

INTRODUCTION

A Guide to Good Reasoning provides a complete practical system for evaluating arguments. It also provides an account of how mastery of this system can contribute to the broader goal of becoming a good reasoner—the goal of becoming intellectually honest, critically reflective and empirically inquisitive. But the core of the book is the practical system, and your professor can—and probably will—use the system as one important way of measuring your performance. This supplement aims to provide a handy tool to which you can easily refer as you begin to master it.

Except for the sample answers and the section that discusses the Web, everything in the manual can be found in the textbook in expanded form; key points are simply consolidated here for ready reference. The first two sections are checklists for clarifying and evaluating; the third provides a real-life application of the system to the World Wide Web; the fourth is a glossary of all key terms in the textbook; and the fifth contains sample answers to all the book's odd exercises.

The Basic Concepts

There are only a handful of ideas that you need to learn in order to have the outline of the whole system firmly in mind:

> Four merits of arguments—truth, logic, conversational relevance, and clarity.
> Two principles for clarifying—loyalty and charity.
> Three procedures for clarifying—streamlining, specifying, and structuring.
> Standard clarifying format.
> The clarifying rule of thumb—"imagine the arguer over your shoulder."
> Standard evaluating format.
> The evaluating rule of thumb—"imagine a reasonable objector over your shoulder."
> Two broad kinds of evidence for truth—inferential and noninferential (the latter including self-evidence and experiential evidence).

Two conditions for good logic—the correct form condition and
(for inductive arguments only) the total evidence condition.
The checklists that follow fill in this outline.

The Key to the System: The Four Merits of Arguments

Although the emphasis in this manual is strictly practical, there is one
piece of theory that you must grasp from the start if you are to have any
practical success: the four merits of arguments. They are as follows:

1. ***TRUE PREMISES***—the premises *fit with the world.*

2. ***GOOD LOGIC***—the conclusion *fits with the evidence.*

   - *Deductive* arguments—the conclusion fits strictly with the
     premises.
   - *Inductive* arguments—the conclusion fits with the premises
     and with the total evidence.

3. ***CONVERSATIONAL RELEVANCE***—the argument *fits with the
   conversation.*

4. ***CLARITY***—*you can tell whether it fits* in the preceding three
   ways.

When you *clarify* an argument, you are introducing more of the fourth
merit, clarity, into the argument. When you *evaluate* an argument, you
are then able to focus entirely on the first three merits. (The first two
merits constitute *soundness*.)

2

SECTION ONE

Checklist for Clarifying Arguments

❑ *BE SURE IT IS AN ARGUMENT*

1. **DOES IT SATISFY THE DEFINITION OF *ARGUMENT*?** A simple argument is a series of statements in which one of the statements is offered as a reason to believe another. A complex argument is a series of simple arguments in which the conclusion to one simple argument is a premise in the next simple argument.

2. **CAN YOU FIND A CONCLUSION?** If you can find a conclusion, it is an argument. If you can't instinctively tell which statement is being supported by the others, here are three tips.

   - *Look for the most controversial statement.* Since arguments typically appeal to plausible premises to support less plausible conclusions, the most controversial statement is usually the conclusion.

   - *Look in the broader context for the question that is being asked.* Since arguments are usually offered to answer some question of interest, the statement that provides the answer to the question is usually the conclusion.

   - *Look for inference indicators.*

BEFORE PREMISES	BEFORE CONCLUSIONS
Since	Therefore
Because	Thus
For	Hence
My reason is	So
On account of	Consequently
The justification is	What this justifies is
Is confirmed by	Confirms
It follows from	It follows that

3. ARE YOU CONFUSING IT WITH A NON-ARGUMENT?

- *Mere assertions* declare something to be true without giving reasons for it.

- *Mere illustrations* provide an example that serves to make clear the meaning of a statement without providing a reason to believe it.

- *Mere explanations* typically move from the unfamiliar to the familiar (unlike arguments) and provide an account of *how* something happens rather than a reason to believe *that* it happens.

❏ *OUTLINE THE ARGUMENT IN STANDARD CLARIFYING FORMAT*

1. Premises numbered above their conclusion.

2. Main conclusion identified as *C.*

3. All conclusions (main conclusion and subconclusions) preceded by ∴ in the left margin.

4. Implicit statements in brackets.

❏ *PARAPHRASE FOR GREATER CLARITY ACCORDING TO TWO PRINCIPLES*

1. **THE PRINCIPLE OF LOYALTY**—paraphrase in a way that remains true to the arguer's intent.

   - Imagine that the arguer is looking over your shoulder.

2. **THE PRINCIPLE OF CHARITY**—paraphrase in a way that makes the arguer as reasonable as possible. This helps you achieve loyalty when the context does not make clear the arguer's intent.

   • Imagine that you uttered the same words under similar circumstances, in order to paraphrase others as you would have them paraphrase you (thus, this is known as the golden rule of paraphrasing).

❏ *STREAMLINE YOUR PARAPHRASE*

1. **PARAPHRASE NON-STATEMENTS** as statements, focusing on expressions such as these:

   • Imperatives that conclude practical reasoning.
   • Rhetorical questions.
   • Fragments.

2. **ELIMINATE DISCOUNTS**—statements offered as not undermining the conclusion (rather than as reasons to believe the conclusion). Some *discount indicators* are:

BACKWARD-POINTING	FORWARD-POINTING
But	In spite of
However	Despite
Nevertheless	Although
Nonetheless	Though
Yet	Regardless of
Still	Notwithstanding

3. **ELIMINATE ATTITUDE INDICATORS** such as "I believe" and "it is doubtful that."

4. **ELIMINATE REPORT INDICATORS** such as "she argued that" and "his view was that."

5. **ELIMINATE INFERENCE INDICATORS** such as "thus" and "since."

6. **ELIMINATE REPETITION**

7. **ELIMINATE WORDINESS**

8. **NEUTRALIZE SLANTED LANGUAGE**

❏ *SPECIFY IN YOUR PARAPHRASE*

1. **AMBIGUITY** should be removed by rewriting the ambiguous statement in an unambiguous way. This will help you avoid the fallacy of equivocation (which results from semantic ambiguity) and the fallacy of amphiboly (which results from syntactic ambiguity. Two strategies for removing ambiguity are these.

   - *The reasonable-premises strategy*—paraphrase the ambiguity so as to make the premises as reasonable as possible. This will usually demonstrate that the logic is defective.

   - *The reasonable-logic strategy*—paraphrase the ambiguity so as to make the logic successful. This will usually result in a clearly false premise.

2. **GENERALITY** should be removed when it results in a fallacy of ambiguity.

3. **VAGUENESS** should not tempt you to accept a slippery slope argument or an argument from the heap.

4. **EMPTINESS** should not be introduced into your paraphrase when you can, instead, provide information from the context.

❑ *STRUCTURE YOUR PARAPHRASE*

1. **IDENTIFY THE LOGICAL FORM** of the argument. Most arguments will fit one of the following forms.

DEDUCTIVE FORMS

Conjunction
1. P
2. Q
∴ C. P and Q

Double negation
1. P
∴ C. Not not P

1. Not not P.
∴ C. P

Repetition
1. P
∴ C. P

Simplification
1. P and Q
∴ C. P

Affirming the antecedent
1. If P then Q.
2. P
∴ C. Q

Denying the consequent
1. If P then Q.
2. Not Q.
∴ C. Not P.

Fallacy of affirming consequent (invalid)
1. If P then Q.
2. Q
∴ C. P

Fallacy of denying antecedent (invalid)
1. If P then Q.
2. Not P.
∴ C. Not Q.

Transitivity of implication
1. If P then Q.
2. If Q then R.
∴ C. If P then R.

Affirming an exclusive alternative
1. P or Q only one.
2. P
∴ C. Not Q.

DeMorgan's laws
1. Not (P or Q).
∴ C. Not P and not Q.

1. Not (P and Q).
∴ C. Not P or not Q.

Disjunction
1. P
∴ C. P or Q

Either-or dilemma
1. P or Q.
2. If P then R.
3. If Q then R.
C. R

1. P or Q.
2. If P then R.
3. If Q then S.
∴ C. R or S.

1. P or Q.
2. If R then not P.
3. If R then not Q.
∴ C. Not R.

1. P or Q.
2. If R then not P.
3. If S then not Q.
∴ C. Not R or not S.

Fallacy of affirming an alternative (invalid)
1. P or Q.
2. P
∴ C. Not Q.

If-then dilemma
1. If T, then P or Q.
2. If P then R.
3. If Q then R.
∴ C. If T, then R.

Process of elimination
1. P or Q
2. Not P
C. Q

1. P or Q
2. Not Q
C. P

1. P or Q or R
2. Not P
C. Q or R

1. P or Q or R
2. Not P
3. Not Q
C. R

Singular version of any of the above

Singular categorical argument
1. All F are G.
2. A is F.
C. A is

7

INDUCTIVE FORMS

Frequency argument
1. *n* of *F* are *G* (where *n* is a frequency >.5 and <1, i.e., more than half, less than all).
2. *A* is *F*.
∴ C. *A* is *G*.

1. *n* of *F* are *G.* (where *n* is a frequency <.5 and >0, i.e., less than half, more than none)
2. *A* is *F*.
∴ C. *A* is not *G*.

Inductive generalization
1. *n* of sampled *F* are *G.* (Where n is *any* frequency, including 0 and 1.)
∴ C. *n* (+ or - *m*) of *F* are *G*.

Argument from analogy
1. *A* is *F* and *G.*
2. *B* is *F.*
∴ C. *B* is *G.*

Explanatory argument
1.   If *P* then *Q*.
2.   *Q*
∴ C. *P*

2. **TRANSLATE STYLISTIC VARIANTS** for constants into standard constants.

3. **MATCH THE WORDING** in your paraphrase when the same name, predicate, or statement is expressed in different words.

❏ *SUPPLY THE IMPORTANT IMPLICIT STATEMENTS*, in accordance with all of the above.

SECTION TWO

Checklist for Evaluating Arguments

❑ *OUTLINE YOUR EVALUATION IN STANDARD EVALUATION FORMAT.*

1. Heading: EVALUATION

2. Subheading: TRUTH. For each premise, state whether you judge it to be true, and provide your defense of that judgment. If a reasonable objector would have an objection, state the objection and respond to it.

3. Subheading: LOGIC. State whether you judge the logic to be successful and provide your defense of that judgment.

4. Subheading: SOUNDNESS. State whether you judge the argument to be sound; if and only if it is not sound, state whether this is owing to a problem with a premise or with the logic.

5. Subheading (optional): CONVERSATIONAL RELEVANCE. If and only if the argument is flawed in this way, state whether it commits the fallacy of begging the question or missing the point, and explain how.

6. If the argument is complex, include each of these four subheadings for each simple argument, indicating in each case which simple argument you are evaluating with the heading **EVALUATION OF THE ARGUMENT TO N.**

❑ *FOLLOW THE "REASONABLE OBJECTOR" PRINCIPLE IN WRITING YOUR EVALUATION*

Imagine that looking over your shoulder is a reasonable person who disagrees with your evaluation, and whom you must convince. This **REASONABLE OBJECTOR** has roughly the same evidence that you have, and possesses the intellectual virtues of honesty, critical reflection, and inquiry.

❑ *BEWARE OF ARGUMENTS COMMITTING MOTIVE-BASED FALLACIES*

1. Pay special attention to arguments that tend to promote motives other than wanting to know the truth about the question at issue; they commit fallacies such as:

- *Ad hominem* fallacy
- Fallacy of appealing to authority
- Fallacy of appealing to sympathy
- Fallacy of appealing to consequences

2. These arguments are likely to be lacking at least one of the four merits of arguments. Focus your written evaluation on the merit that it lacks, not on the motives it promotes.

❑ *IDENTIFY ARGUMENT-BASED FALLACIES IN YOUR EVALUATION*

1. **CLARITY**-based fallacies.

- Fallacy of equivocation—identify under the logic heading if you use the reasonable-premises strategy of paraphrasing, under the truth heading if you use the reasonable-logic strategy of paraphrasing.
- Fallacy of amphiboly—same as above.

- Slippery slope fallacy—identify typically under the logic heading.
- Fallacy of argument from the heap—identify typically under the logic heading.

2. **TRUTH-based fallacies.** Instead of identifying fallacies, it is typically better to focus under truth on any specific reason the premise might not be true. Exceptions: the fallacies of equivocation and amphiboly may be included when you have paraphrased using the reasonable-logic strategy; and the fallacy of *non causa pro causa* may be included when, in an indirect argument, the if-then premise is found to be at fault due to a false secondary assumption.

3. **DEDUCTIVE LOGIC-based fallacies.**

- Fallacy of affirming the consequent
- Fallacy of denying the antecedent
- Fallacy of affirming an alternative
- Fallacy of composition
- Fallacy of division

4. **INDUCTIVE LOGIC-based fallacies.** In inductive arguments, it is usually better to show specifically how the inductive argument fails to meet the total evidence condition than to identify the fallacy.

- Fallacy of hasty generalization
- Fallacy of false analogy
- Fallacy of *post hoc ergo propter hoc*

5. **CONVERSATIONAL RELEVANCE-based fallacies.**

- Fallacy of missing the point
- Fallacy of begging the question

❑ *ANSWER THE QUESTION* "ARE THE PREMISES TRUE?" *FOR EACH PREMISE AND DEFEND YOUR ANSWER.*

1. STATE YOUR ASSESSMENT of the truth-value of each premise in terms of epistemic probability, using terms such as certainly true, probably true, can't decide, probably false, certainly false.

2. PROVIDE YOUR STRONGEST REASON IN FAVOR OF YOUR ASSESSMENT, but do not simply paraphrase the premise or its negation. Here are some tips for different situations:

   TYPES OF EVIDENCE

   - *Inferential evidence*—appeal to well-supported beliefs of yours.

   - *Self-evidence*—appeal to your understanding of the meaning of the terms.

   - *Experiential evidence*—appeal to your sensory experiences. If true, show the following conditions hold:
     - The circumstances of the observation make your experience a reliable one.
     - There is no reason to doubt your memory of the experience.
     - The prior probability of the premise is reasonably high.
     If false, show the opposite for at least one of these conditions.

   - *Evidence from authoritative sources*—appeal to reliable sources (this is a kind of experiential evidence). If true, show the following conditions hold:
     - The circumstances of the observation make the source a reliable one.
     - The prior probability of the premise is reasonably high. .
     If false, show the opposite for at least one of these conditions.

TYPES OF PREMISES

- *Both-and premise*—if one part is almost certainly false, it is almost certainly false; if both are almost certainly true, it is almost certainly true. Otherwise do this:
    - Multiply the epistemic probabilities of each part, **OR**
    - If the truth of one part would affect the probability of the second part, when you multiply the probabilities of the two parts you should use for the second part its probability *on the assumption that the first one is true.*
  Defend your judgment by indicating the evidence regarding both parts and, if necessary, by explaining the math.

- *Either-or premise*—if both alternatives are almost certainly false, it is almost certainly false; if one is almost certainly true, it is almost certainly true. Otherwise do this:
    - Add the epistemic probabilities of each alternative, **AND**
    - Subtract the probability that both alternatives are simultaneously true.
  Defend your judgment by indicating the evidence regarding both alternatives and, if necessary, by explaining the math.

- *If-then premise*—if the if-clause is almost certainly true and the then-clause is almost certainly false, then it is almost certainly false. This can be defended by providing the evidence regarding both clauses or, if it is a universal statement, by a truth counterexample. Otherwise, do this:
    - Identify the unstated secondary assumptions that are intended to link the if-clause to the then-clause.
    - If the if-then clause is true, show that the most plausible secondary assumptions are true. If it is false, show that at least one of them is false.

- *Premise about sampling*—samples are often misunderstood, producing a false premise. The more hidden the property, the greater the opportunity for misunderstanding. (Human beliefs and desires, for example, are hidden, and relying on human reports of their own beliefs and desires can be misleading.)

3. **RESPOND TO THE MOST REASONABLE OBJECTION TO YOUR ASSESSMENT**, if there is one.

❏ *ANSWER THE QUESTION "IS THE LOGIC GOOD?" FOR EACH SIMPLE ARGUMENT AND DEFEND YOUR ANSWER.*

DEDUCTIVE ARGUMENTS
The question "Is the logic good?" should be taken to mean "Do the premises guarantee the conclusion?"

1. **STATE YOUR ASSESSMENT** of the argument's logic, by saying either that it is "valid" or "invalid." A valid argument satisfies the *correct form condition* for deductive arguments, that is, it possesses a form such that it is impossible for an argument with that form to have true premises and a false conclusion; an invalid one does not satisfy this condition.

2. **DEFEND YOUR ASSESSMENT** of the argument's logic.
   If valid, state the name of the valid form, such as the following:

- Repetition
- Conjunction
- Simplification
- Affirming the antecedent.
- Denying the consequent.
- Transitivity of implication
- Process of elimination
- Affirming an exclusive alternative
- DeMorgan's law
- Either-or dilemma
- If-then dilemma
- Singular version of any of the above
- Singular categorical syllogism

If invalid, state the name of the fallacy (if there is a name) and provide a validity counterexample, which requires two steps:

- Extract the form that the argument depends upon.
- Provide a new argument in that form that has obviously true premises and an obviously false conclusion.

INDUCTIVE ARGUMENTS

The question "Is the logic good" should be taken to mean, "Do the premises make probable the conclusion?"

1. **STATE YOUR ASSESSMENT** of the argument's logic by saying where it is on the continuum from "very strong" to "very weak" to "no support at all." Two conditions must be satisfied.

   - *Correct form condition*—necessary for any strength at all.
   - *Total evidence condition*—formulated differently for each form of inductive argument. Assuming the correct form condition is satisfied, the degree to which the argument satisfies this condition determines the argument's degree of logical strength.

2. **DEFEND YOUR ASSESSMENT** of the argument's logic. If it satisfies the correct form condition, say so; then address how well the argument satisfies the version of the total evidence condition that applies to it.

   - *Frequency arguments*—two parts to the total evidence condition:
     (1) The higher the stated frequency, the greater the strength the argument can have (but its strength cannot exceed that frequency).
     (2) Background evidence can prevent the argument from being as strong as the frequency stated in the first premise.

   - *Inductive generalizations*—two parts to the total evidence condition:

(1) The sample must be large enough. If the property is all-or-none, then a sample of one is usually enough for a logically strong argument. If it is not all-or-none, then a randomly selected sample of 1,000 with a margin of error of 3 percent can provide a logically strong argument.

(2) The sample must be randomly selected. Be especially wary of grab sampling, snowball sampling, self-selected sampling, and dirty sampling.

- *Arguments from analogy*—two parts to the total evidence condition:
  (1) The basic similarity must be relevant—it must count in favor of the inferred similarity.
  (2) The dissimilarities must be irrelevant—any dissimilarity between the two analogs must not make the basic analog a better candidate for the inferred property.

- *Explanatory arguments*—two parts to the total evidence condition:
  (1) The observable outcome must be sufficiently improbable. This means that you should reject unfalsifiable explanations, favor precise outcomes, favor outcomes for which no explanation already exists, and favor outcomes that would falsify alternative explanations.
  (2) The explanation must be sufficiently probable. This means that you should favor frequency, favor explanations that make sense, favor simplicity, look for coincidence as an alternative explanation, and look for deception as an alternative explanation.

❑ *ANSWER THE QUESTION "IS THE ARGUMENT SOUND?"*
FOR EACH SIMPLE ARGUMENT AND, IF IT IS UNSOUND,
DEFEND YOUR ANSWER.

1. STATE YOUR ASSESSMENT of the argument's soundness. It is
    sound if and only if the premises are true and the logic is good.
    Qualify your assessment, when necessary, to reflect the weakest
    thing you have already said about the premises or the logic.

2. DEFEND YOUR ASSESSMENT of the argument's soundness if and
    only if the argument is unsound by concisely stating where you
    have identified the problem—for example, "probably unsound
    because premise 2 is probably false" or "moderately unsound
    because the logic is moderately weak."

❑ *CONSIDER THE QUESTION "IS THE ARGUMENT*
CONVERSATIONALLY RELEVANT?" FOR EACH SIMPLE
ARGUMENT AND, IF IT IS NOT, ANSWER THE QUESTION
AND DEFEND YOUR ANSWER.

1. STATE YOUR ASSESSMENT that the argument is not
    conversationally relevant if it is not.

2. DEFEND YOUR ASSESSMENT by identifying the fallacy it commits
    and explain how it does so. The two fallacies of conversational
    relevance are these:

    - Fallacy of missing the point.
    - Fallacy of begging the question.

SECTION THREE

Good Reasoning and the Web[1]

Michael Gorman, writing in the *Library Journal*, describes the World Wide Web as follows:

> The net is like a huge vandalized library. Someone has destroyed the catalog and removed the front matter, indexes, etc., from hundreds of thousands of books and torn and scattered what remains.... The net is even worse than a vandalized library because thousands of additional unorganized fragments are added daily by the myriad cranks, sages, and persons with time on their hands who launch their unfiltered messages into cyberspace."[2]

Culture critic Wayne Miller of UCLA likens the Web, alternatively, to a gigantic pamphlet distribution center. Each Web address is like a slot in a pamphlet rack, its content constantly and unpredictably changing. And, like pamphlets, Web pages are easy for anyone with a message to publish and even easier for anyone with a fleeting interest to pick up—but not to evaluate.

I am writing this toward the end of 1998. The Web is evolving so rapidly that many of the specifics in this section will quickly become dated. But the general problem noted by Gorman and Miller is likely to remain—namely, anyone can publish anything on the Web and thereby gain an audience and an aura of respectability. You can do it even if you are in prison—Charles Manson has his own Web site. But it is easier if you are on parole. You need access only to a computer with a modem (borrow a friend's, use one at the local library or copy center, or buy one for $399), which needs to be connected by phone to an Internet service

---

[1] I am especially grateful to UCLA's Michael Cohen, Mike Franks, Wayne Miller, and Evan Nisonson for their help with this section.

[2] Michael Gorman, "The Corruption of Cataloging," *Library Journal*, September 15, 1995, p. 34.

provider (another $10 to $15 per month—though some providers are experimenting with free, advertiser-supported, access). If the Internet service provider does not provide free space for your Web site (many do), simply connect to www.geocities.com, and they will provide you with free space. It helps if you know HTML (hypertext markup language), but it isn't required. You do need to be able to use a computer keyboard. Unlike traditional print publication (but more like pamphleteering), there is no staff to check your facts, no editor to examine your work, nobody to sign off on its accuracy before it is released.

The good news is that, for all the same reasons, the Web is dramatically enhancing our ability to communicate. Indeed, there is so much of positive value on the Web that it is already an indispensable resource. Web expert Mike Franks, author of the *Internet Publishing Handbook,*[3] writes this in a recent e-mail:

> The Web can be a great democratizing force, giving everyone the chance to have a say. And the lack of an editor doesn't automatically result in garbage. Remember that some faculty have commented that when students know their papers will go on the Web, they do a better job.

How to begin to make sense of it? In this section of the manual, I provide some specific suggestions to help you make a start toward reasoning well when you make use of the Web.

Of the four merits of arguments, my comments have very little to do with *logic* on the Web—affirming the antecedent is just as valid on the Web as it is in *Newsweek*, and false analogies are just as logically weak. Nor do my comments bear significantly on *conversational relevance* or *clarity*—as with logic, what is said in the textbook about these topics can be applied without difficulty to the Web. What does merit close attention, however, is reliance upon the Web in support of your judgment about the *truth of premises*. This section, then, can be seen as an appendix to the book's Part Four: Evaluating the Truth of Premises.

Recall that one important sort of experiential evidence, as described in Chapter 9 (beginning on page 228), is *what authorities have reported,*

---

[3] Mike Franks, *Internet Publishing Handbook* (NY: Addison-Wesley Publishing Co., 1995), also on the Web in its entirety at http://www.sscnet.ucla. edu/ssc/franks/ book/.

where an authority is defined as anyone who is presumed to be in a better position than you to know the truth about the premise in question. This is where the Web comes in, and it is what we will focus on. When should you presume that a Web source is in a better position than you to know the truth about some question? No source of information comes with a guarantee of reliability—even our five senses, as we have noted, can betray us—but what sorts of things suggest that a Web source is *probably* reliable?

Consider the Site's Neighborhood

You can learn a few useful things if you take a look at the site's address and its front yard. Look, for example, at the *extension* of the *domain name* of the site. This is typically a three-letter term that occurs after the second dot after *www*. The domain name for McGraw-Hill Higher Education's Web site, www.mhhe.com, for example, is *mhhe.com*, and its extension is *com*.

The most reliable information is likely to be found in the domain *gov*; these are tightly controlled sites used by U.S. government organizations to post official data, forms, and policies and procedures. For example, take a look at the IRS Web site, www.irs.ustreas.gov. "Most reliable" doesn't mean "perfectly reliable," of course. A site that presents the government's position on a controversial issue can be trusted...to be the government's position. Also, bear in mind that government sites are prime targets for hackers—who have invaded, among others, the FBI, CIA, Department of Commerce, and Department of Justice sites. If you have special concerns about this, you can visit a site dedicated to tracking significant hacks, both governmental and otherwise: www.2600.com/hacked_pages/.

Org and *edu* are two domain extensions that also tend (with emphasis on "tend") to be reliable, though they are a notch or two below *gov*. *Org* was established for non-profit organizations—the NAACP, for example, is at www.naacp.org, and the American Psychological Association is at www.apa.org. Non-profits, of course, sometimes have a strong interest in getting you to see things their way, so be on the alert for sites with spin. And, alas, registration for this extension has not been tightly controlled, so there is no guarantee that an *org* site is not angling for a profit.

Edu sites, on the other hand, are used by educational institutions—note, for example, the home page of my institution, `www.ucla.edu`. University sites are less tightly controlled than either *gov* or *org* sites, since faculty—who can be almost impossible to fire—can be almost impossible to control. Faculty, then, tend to put whatever they wish on their Web sites. Since they also tend to put whatever they wish into their lectures, you can trust their Web sites about as much as their lectures. That is, I hasten to add, you can usually trust them—but be ready for a little rhetoric and a few idiosyncrasies. *Edu* sites, however, include much more than university business and academic content. Nobody tells UCLA multimedia specialist Michael Cohen, for example, that he can't post his cartoons on `http://www.humnet.ucla.edu/hcf/staff/mcohen/chuckle.html`. And be prepared for plenty of student pages in *edu* territory, since universities often provide their students with free space. A tilde (that is, "~") in the address often indicates a page that is more or less autonomous—for example, `www.ucla.edu/~name`. You should apply to these pages, of course, whatever criteria are normally appropriate for judging the reliability of your fellow students.

There are a few extensions that are less familiar—*net*, for example, is a seldom seen extension used by those who provide network services (though sometimes even these service providers will rent out *net* space to others who may be less trustworthy). And more domain extensions are slated soon to appear. But by far the most common extension is *com*. This is really where the vast pamphlet market exists, and where the greatest care must be exercised. For judging sites with *com* addresses, I refer you to suggestions later in this section.

You can, of course, tell a little bit more by looking past the address and checking out the front yard. But only a little bit. You should worry about a site that reflects no intelligence in its design. But some sites with nothing but boring text are chock-full of valuable information, while others with elegant graphics are useless. Take note, if you have the time, of `www.whitehouse.net`. The domain name is encouraging, and the design is gorgeous. You seem to have arrived at the president's home page...and then you begin to notice that the White House in the photo is sometimes pink, sometimes green, and that unfamiliar pictures sometimes appear over the names of the president and vice president, and...um...isn't that a Jolly Roger rather than the American flag? Don't count on doing research here—it's a gentle spoof.

Consider the Site's Reputation

Many sites come with the equivalent of letters of recommendation. The letters arrive in at least two forms. First, if other reputable Web sites link to a site, that is an indicator of reliability. You can find out which sites link to another site by going to a search engine—say, AltaVista (at `www.altavista.com`), and entering as your search item the full Web address for the site in question. This will produce a list of sites that link to it. The credibility of a site providing facts about AIDS, for example, is greatly enhanced if the list shows that medical centers at Harvard, Berkeley, Johns Hopkins, and UCLA link to it.

As always, however, exercise caution. Letters of recommendation are extremely useful in deciding whether to offer someone a job or admit someone to law school, but they have well-known hazards. Sometimes it is hard to know exactly what a letter writer means (let's see—when she writes "I recommend this student with no qualifications whatsoever," is it the recommendation or the student that has no qualifications)? It can likewise be hard to know what a link means. Try the AltaVista technique, for example, with the "Aids Facts" site at the address `http://147.129.1.10/library/lib2/AIDSFACTS.html`. There are about two dozen links to it, and many of them seem quite respectable. But, alas, if you check them out you will find that they link to it as an example of an unreliable Web site! (Try it yourself and you'll see why.)

A second type of recommendation is more direct. There are several services that evaluate Web sites and advertise the ones that pass muster. When you use sites recommended by them, you are, in effect, relying upon the service as a sort of editorial board. Some of these services (LookSmart and NetGuide, for example) send a logo to the Webmaster so that their seal of approval can be seen by all; but you can also go directly to the services' own sites and link from there to approved sites of interest to you. Three reputable services are:

Argus Clearinghouse	`www.clearinghouse.net`
LookSmart	`www.looksmart.com`
NetGuide	`www.netguide.com`

A service that you should find especially useful if you are working on a term paper is provided by Infomine at `http://infomine.ucr.edu/main.html`; it is designed by university librarians as a guide to the most valuable and dependable sites for research purposes. A similar, though far less discriminating, service is provided by Yahoo at `www.yahoo.com`. Yahoo maintains a team of reviewers who catalog meritorious sites. When you do a Yahoo search, you do get the indiscriminate list of thousands of sites that make use of the terms you have entered, but sometimes you get more. If their team has already personally cataloged your term, Yahoo first provides you with "category" matches that it has found, and within these categories are their approved sites.

Just as some letter writers are known for praising everyone as the greatest law school prospect since F. Lee Bailey, some of these rating services can be easy to please. The best *looking* seal of approval says *Top 5% Best of the Web*. It is awarded by Point.com, an outfit which has been criticized for relying on untrained volunteers, following ill-defined criteria, and having no clue to how many Web sites actually exist—and thus no clue to how many would actually make up the top 5%. (See, for example, the *WebReview* article about their service at `http://webreview.com`, titled "Get Rich Quick! Rate Web Sites!") Their logo on a site, according to their critics, means that somebody or other liked the site for some reason or other. But you don't need to be told that.

Consider the Site's Author

A recent New Yorker cartoon shows a dog sitting at a computer, thinking, "On the Internet, nobody knows you're a dog." It's not always easy to discover the identity, the credentials, or even the species of a Web site's author. If it is clearly an institutional site—say, within the *gov* or *org* domain—this may be irrelevant, since the institution is taking responsibility for the site. Nor do the identity or credentials of the author especially matter if the site is interactive and you are simply scouting for some man-on-the-street impressions of a movie (as with the Internet Movie DataBase at `www.imdb.com`), or of a book or recording (as with Amazon.com at `www.amazon.com`). But when it is an individual's site and your use of the site's information calls for accuracy and objectivity, it is important to know about the author.

The worst case is when there is no mention of the author and no way of finding out (for example, no link with additional information, or no e-mail address). Here I can offer only two suggestions. First, you can go to `www.internic.net`; in the search window that is provided, enter the address in question and it will tell you to whom it is registered (including e-mail address, mailing address, and phone number). This works, however, only for the top level of the address, that is, for the part of the address that ends with the extension, such as www.aol.com. If the address of the site in question continues beyond that level (and most of them do), you will then have to e-mail the person to whom the top-level address is registered, in effect asking the landlord for information about the tenant. If that doesn't work and you are willing to put more effort into the inquiry, try sending an e-mail to "webmaster" at the domain name (for example, for McGraw-Hill Higher Education, try webmaster@mhhe.com) and ask for the name, credentials (and species) of the author in question. Once you do have this information about the author, then you're no worse off than with any other medium.

Consider the Site's Content

When it comes to the content of the Web site, the generic rules introduced in the textbook directly apply. The author's claims must have a reasonably high prior probability (that is, they must be reasonably probable *independent* of their appearance on the site); otherwise, you should not believe them *solely* on the basis of the site. This criterion applies to any medium, of course. But the Web is a magnet for those with preposterous claims. You may wish to examine the site at www.d-b.net/dti. No site could possibly look more professional. And it trumpets endorsements from apparently reputable sources such as the *BioScience Journal*. But something is amiss. They make this claim for their company: "Since March 18, 1997, we've helped 62,554 lives come into existence. No other cloning company comes close!" Then you might notice the company name on the masthead—"Clones R Us." Other sources are needed before we take this site's word for it.

The Web is also a magnet for those with a conflict of interest. It can be a very good sign if a site links to other sites that express different points of views. But it can be a very bad sign if the site extols the virtues of a service or product and then provides you with a link or an 800 number for ordering it. An excellent example of this is found at www.smartbasic.com/glos.news/1.listening.to.5htp.html. On this site, Charles Davidson (no credentials provided) offers a highly technical and scholarly-sounding survey of the effects of a compound called 5-HTP, which, he suggests, can work to suppress appetite, induce sleep, moderate PMS, and alleviate depression. After concluding with 27 impressive bibliographic entries, we find the following banner: CONTACT US TO PLACE ORDERS, SPEAK WITH CUSTOMER SERVICE OR RECEIVE QUOTES FOR THE LOWEST WORLD-WIDE SHIPPING RATES. The link for placing orders follows, accompanied by an 800 number and a fax number, should that prove more convenient.

Consider the Site's Timeliness

There are instances when you should be especially alert to when the information on the site was last updated. This doesn't matter, of course, if the site offers the text of Dickens's *Oliver Twist* or baseball statistics for the 1927 Yankees. But in many other cases it matters very much. The Dow Jones Industrial Average of two days ago, for example, is not of much value to anyone. In such cases, the absence of a date is a reason for concern. And the mere presence of a date is not necessarily a reason to relax, unless it is clear that the date indicates when the information on the site was last revised. Dates on Web sites can point to when the site was created, when the document itself was originally created, or when the site was last revised. Make sure you can tell the difference.

If you can't tell the difference, there are still two simple tests you can run. First, some browsers will tell you when a site was last modified. In Netscape, for example, select the "View" option and then select "Document Information." A recent date there, after "last modified," doesn't guarantee that the information you care about was modified recently, but an old date guarantees that it wasn't. Second, try out several of the site's links. If some of them are dead, then the site is probably comatose.

A Note on Logic

Although our focus has been on truth, there is one important point about logic to bear in mind (a point also made on page 391 of the textbook). Surveys are a popular feature of Web sites. The ESPN site asks who is the NFL's best quarterback, while CNN's site asks whether the president should be impeached. In many cases there is instant gratification—you are told immediately the current results of the balloting, as a sort of reward for voting. Every such survey should be labeled with a large warning: GENERALIZE WITH CARE. The sample is almost always *large* enough for you to generalize to the views of the population at large— recall that for a randomly selected sample, 1,000 are enough for a 3 percent margin of error. But the sample is almost never *randomly selected*. It is self-selected. Thus, it represents the views of those who can afford access to the Web, have sufficient education to make use of the Web, have an interest in the topic of the Web site—and, more specifically, those who have an interest in knowing what people like them think about the question in the survey. My generalization from the Web surveys that I have sampled is that they are often useful for entertainment, but seldom useful for generalization.

SECTION FOUR

Glossary

Ad hominem *fallacy*—a motive-based fallacy that rejects a view by irrelevantly drawing attention to something undesirable about a person who holds it, rather than drawing attention to the merits of the view itself. It takes advantage of our desire to distance ourselves from undesirables. Often a diversionary tactic rather than an argument.

Affirming an exclusive alternative—a valid argument form, as follows:
      1. *P* or *Q* and only one.
      2. *P*
∴   *C*. Not *Q*.
Historically known as *modus ponendo tollens*, Latin for "the method of affirming in order to deny."

Affirming the antecedent—a valid deductive form, as follows:
      1. If *P* then *Q*.
      2. *P*
∴   *C*. *Q*
Also known as *modus ponens,* which is Latin for "the method (or mode, from *modus*) of affirming (or propounding, from *ponens*)."

Alternative—a statement connected to another by *or*. Also known as *disjunct*.

Ambiguity—occurs when an expression has more than one possible meaning and it is not clear which meaning is intended.

Analogs—the two things (or classes of things) that are said to be similar in an argument from analogy.

Antecedent—the if-clause of an if-then statement.

29

Argument—a series of statements in which at least one of the statements is offered as reason to believe another.

Argument from analogy—argument that asserts that because two items are the same in one respect, they are the same in another respect. They can be represented by this form:
1. *A* is *F* and *G*.
2. *B* is *F.*
∴   *C. B* is *G.*

Argument-based fallacy—fallacy that reflects a specific flaw in one of the four merits of an argument: its clarity, the truth of its premises, its logic, or its conversational relevance.

Attitude indicator—indicates the arguer's attitude of either belief or disbelief toward a statement. *I believe that* and *I deny that* are examples.

Authority—someone who is presumed to be in a better position than you to know the truth about a statement. This superiority may be due to either special ability (as with a scientist or expert) or special access (as with an eyewitness or a journalist).

Background argument—an argument that shows that the inferred similarity (of an analogical argument) follows from the basic similarity, that is, an argument that shows that the basic similarity is relevant.

Basic analog—in an argument from analogy, the item that we are presumably more familiar with, which is presumably known to have both the basic and the inferred similarities.

Basic similarity—in an argument from analogy, the property that the two analogs share, presumably without controversy.

Both-and argument—one of a loosely defined group of deductive arguments that have a both-and statement as a premise.

Both-and statement—a statement of the form *P and Q*. Also called a *conjunction*, though we are reserving this term for a deductive form.

Categorical statement—a statement of the form *All F are G, No F are G, Some F are G,* or *Some F are not G*.

Categorical syllogism—one of a family of deductive arguments, some valid and others invalid, each with three categorical statements—two as premises, one as conclusion.

Clarifying--ensuring that the argument is expressed as clearly as possible, so it is as easy as possible to tell whether the premises are true, whether the logic is good, and whether the argument is relevant to the conversation.

Clear argument—an argument in which it is possible to tell whether the premises are true, whether the logic is good, and whether the argument is conversationally relevant.

Complex argument—a series of two or more simple arguments, in which the conclusion of one argument serves as a premise for the next. Complex arguments can be made up of any number of simple arguments, and thus may have any number of subconclusions.

Conclusion--the statement in an argument for which the reasons are offered. Each simple argument has exactly one conclusion.

Confidence level—the logical strength of the argument; the frequency with which the conclusion would be true if the premises were true.

Confirmation bias—our natural tendency to look for outcomes that support our preferred explanation rather than those that might also falsify the alternatives.

Conjunction—a valid deductive form, as follows:
1. P
2. Q
∴ C. *P* and *Q*

The term is also sometimes used for a both-and statement.

Consequent—the then-clause of an if-then statement.

Conservation shortcut—preserving previously adopted beliefs as a shortcut in reasoning. This can be helpful but is not always supported by the evidence.

Content—the part of the argument that can vary without varying the argument's logical form. It can be made up of statements, names, or predicates. In a description of an argument's form, the place-holders—such as *P* and *Q*—that indicate where the content can vary are termed variables.

Conversational implication--what the speaker or writer wants the audience to believe, over and above the literal meanings of the words that are expressed. These implications are drawn on the basis of broader customs that we all follow that govern the use of certain sorts of expressions under certain circumstances.

Conversationally relevant argument—an argument that is appropriate to the conversation, or the context, that gives rise to it; it does not miss the point or presuppose something that is in question in the conversation.

Correct form condition—the logical requirement on any argument that it exemplify some correct form (that its conclusion fits with its premises). Correct deductive form is sufficient for deductive validity. But correct inductive form is sufficient for inductive strength if and only if it is paired with satisfaction of the total evidence condition.

Critical reflection—asking what the arguments are for what you believe, and whether those arguments are sound, clear, and relevant.

Declarative function—the function of conveying information. An example of a sentence with this function is *Eleanor Roosevelt was one of the most influential First Ladies in history.*

Deductive argument—an argument in which the premises are intended to guarantee, or make certain, the conclusion. To determine whether

the logic of a deductive argument is successful, a good rule of thumb
is to ask questions such as these:
>Do the premises guarantee the conclusion?
>
>If the premises were true, would that make the conclusion
>certain?

Alternatively termed an *apodictic* or *demonstrative* argument.

DeMorgan's laws—valid deductive forms, as follows:
>1. Not (*P* or *Q*).
>
>∴   *C*. Not *P* and not *Q*.
>
>1. Not (*P* and *Q*).
>
>∴   *C*. Not *P* or not *Q*.

Denying the consequent—a valid deductive form, as follows:
>1. If *P* then *Q*.
>2. Not *Q*.
>
>∴   *C*. Not *P*.

Also known as *modus tollens*, which is Latin for "the method of
denying."

Dilemma—a valid deductive form that points out the consequences,
whether good or bad, of two inevitable alternatives. The word comes
from the Greek words *di*, for *two*, and *lemma*, for *proposition*.
Dilemmas come in two varieties: either-or dilemmas and, less
common, if-then dilemmas.

Dirty sampling—the contamination—usually unintentional—of a sample
by the sampling process itself. This is a failure of randomness. In a
randomly selected sample, exactly the relevant variations of the
population are proportionately represented. Introducing
contamination is introducing a relevant variation that is not in the
population.

Discount—a statement the arguer offers as *not undermining* the
conclusion. Discounts are typically neither premises nor
conclusions, and should usually not be included in your clarification.

Discount indicator—a term that indicates a nonsupportive, or adversarial, relationship between statements rather than a supportive one. *But* and *despite* are examples. Sometimes also called *adversative.*

Disjunction—a valid deductive form, as follows:

        1. *P*

∴   *C. P* or *Q*

The term is sometimes also used for an either-or statement.

Double negation—a valid deductive form, as follows:

1. *P*	1. Not not *P*.
∴ *C.* Not not *P.*	∴ *C. P*

Educated ignorance defense—defense of your judgment that an if-then premise is false even though you cannot tell which secondary assumption is at fault (thus, it reflects ignorance); it can be a reasonable defense only if your evidence for the truth of the if-clause and for the falsity of the then-clause is especially and uncontroversially strong (thus, the defense is educated).

Either-or arguments—a loosely defined group of arguments that have an either-or premise. Also called *disjunctive syllogisms.*

Either-or dilemma—a valid dilemma that begins with an either-or premise. The most common forms are these:

        1. *P* or *Q.*

        2. If *P* then *R.*

        3. If *Q* then *R.*

∴   *C. R*

        1. *P* or *Q.*

        2. If *P* then *R.*

        3. If *Q* then *S.*

∴   *C. R* or *S.*

1. P or Q.
2. If R then not P.
3. If R then not Q.
∴ C. Not R.

1. P or Q.
2. If R then not P.
3. If S then not Q.
∴ C. Not R or not S.

Either-or statement—a statement of the form P or Q. Also sometimes called a *disjunction*.

Elliptical ambiguity—semantic ambiguity in which lack of clarity regarding the meaning is due to an expression that has been omitted.

Empirical inquiry—seeking out new evidence from the world around you to better answer your questions.

Empty—a statement that in a normal context would have clear referents for all its terms, but is in a context that provides the audience with no idea of what at least one of its terms refers to.

Enthymeme—an argument with an implicit premise or conclusion. This word comes from the Greek roots *en* for *in* and *thumos* for *mind*; an enthymeme is an argument that leaves a premise or conclusion behind, *in the mind*. For the purposes of clarifying and evaluating, the implicit statements should be considered just as much a part of an enthymematic argument as the explicit ones.

Epistemic—having to do with knowledge.

Epistemic probability—the likelihood that a statement is true, given the total evidence available to you—that is, given all of your background beliefs and experiences. This is the notion of probability that should be used in your evaluation of premises. To say there that a premise is *probably true* is, then, just to say that you have fairly good evidence for its truth.

Exclamatory function—the function of expressing emotion. An example of a sentence with this function is *Oh, to be at the beach this afternoon!*

Exclusivity premise—an either-or premise that includes the notion that only one of the alternatives is true; it has the form *P or Q and only one.*

Experiential evidence—evidence provided by sense experience, that is, that which is seen, heard, touched, smelled, or tasted. It is one kind of noninferential evidence.

Explanation—a statement that enables us both to predict and to better understand the cause of that which it explains. Also termed a *theory* or an *explanatory hypothesis.*

Explanatory argument—an argument which has as its correct form— assuming that *P* is the explanation and *Q* is the observable outcome—the following:

1. If *P* then *Q.*
2. *Q*
∴   C. *P*

The first premise states that the explanation really does enable you to predict the observable outcome—that it really is an *outcome.* The second premise states that the observable outcome has happened— that it has been *observed.* And the argument concludes with the assertion of the explanation. Also called *theoretical arguments, inferences to the best explanation, hypothetico-deductive arguments, transcendental arguments,* and *diagnostic arguments.*

Fallacy—an easy-to-make type of intellectual mistake.

Fallacy of affirming an alternative—an invalid argument form, as follows:

1. *P* or *Q.*
2. *P*
∴   C. Not *Q.*

Fallacy of affirming the consequent—an invalid deductive form, as follows:

1. If P then Q.
2. Q

$\therefore$ C. P

Fallacy of ambiguity—committed by an argument that appears to be successful because of an ambiguous expression that shifts in meaning; the fallacy of equivocation and the fallacy of amphiboly are two varieties.

Fallacy of amphiboly—a fallacy of ambiguity that goes wrong because of syntactic ambiguity.

Fallacy of appealing to authority—a motive-based fallacy that encourages deference to someone else's view when, in fact, those listening to or reading the argument are at least as competent to reason it through as is the presumed authority. Takes advantage of tendency to intellectual timidity. Also known as the *fallacy of argumentum ad verecundiam*, which literally means "appealing to modesty."

Fallacy of appealing to consequences—a motive-based fallacy that directs attention to the practical advantages of a belief rather than the evidence for it. Commonly called *wishful thinking*.

Fallacy of appealing to force—an example of the fallacy of appealing to consequences in which the avoidance of force is the practical advantage of a belief. Also known as the *fallacy of argumentum ad baculum. Baculum* translates to our word *rod*, our closest English word being *bacteria*, which are *rod-shaped*.

Fallacy of appealing to sympathy—a motive-based fallacy that irrelevantly appeals to pity, sympathy, or compassion in support of a conclusion, rather than appealing to considerations that directly bear on the conclusion. Also known as the *fallacy of argumentum ad misericordiam*.

Fallacy of arguing from the heap—the fallacy of mistakenly concluding that because fuzzy borders can take longer to pass, they are impassable.

Fallacy of begging the question—a conversational fallacy that errs by presupposing the answer to what is in question in the conversation. Also known as the *fallacy of petitio principii. Petitio* comes from a word meaning *appeal to,* or *beg,* as in the English word *petition. Principii* is closely related to the English word *principle.* So, *petitio principii* is the fallacy of appealing to a principle that is in question, as though it were already settled.

Fallacy of composition—the mistake of concluding that a property applies to the whole of something because it applies to each of its parts.

Fallacy of denying the antecedent—an invalid deductive form, as follows:

        1. If P then Q.
        2. Not P.
∴ C. Not Q.

Fallacy of division—the mistake of concluding that a property applies to one or more of the parts because it applies to the whole.

Fallacy of equivocation—a fallacy of ambiguity that goes wrong because of semantic ambiguity.

Fallacy of false analogy—the mistake of using an argument from analogy in which the basic similarity is not relevant or in which there are relevant dissimilarities between the basic and inferred analogs. Because this term says nothing about what precisely has gone wrong with the argument, it is better to explain more specifically how it is that some necessary condition for soundness has not been satisfied. Also called the *fallacy of faulty analogy.*

Fallacy of hasty generalization—the mistake of arguing from a sample that is not representative—that is not large enough or randomly selected. It is normally more illuminating if you avoid this term and focus your evaluation on the more specific mistakes made by the argument.

Fallacy of missing the point—a conversational fallacy that errs by answering the wrong question. Also known as the *fallacy of ignoratio elenchi*. *Elenchi* is from a Greek term for *cross-examination*; so, this might be said to be the fallacy of ignoring (*ignoratio*) the question that is being asked (the *elenchi*).

***Fallacy of* non causa pro causa**—the mistake in an indirect argument of relying on a secondary assumption—often implicit—that is false, so that it is really the secondary assumption that should be blamed, not the statement blamed by the arguer. (It literally means that the absurdity is *not caused by the cause that is set forth.*)

Fallacy of singular affirming the consequent—invalid affirming the consequent in which the if-then premise is universal and the conclusion is about a single instance that is encompassed by the universal term.

Fallacy of singular denying the antecedent—invalid denying the antecedent in which the if-then premise is universal and the conclusion is about a single instance that is encompassed by the universal term.

Falsifiability—the requirement that it be possible to specify some observable outcome of an explanation that *could* prove it to be false. This is a way of emphasizing the importance of an improbable outcome. To say that an explanation or an outcome is not falsifiable is to say that *any observation at all* is consistent with the explanation. And it is highly probable that we will have "any observation at all." So, an unfalsifiable explanation fails the improbable outcome test.

Frequency argument—an inductive argument taking one of these forms:
1. n of F are G (where n is a frequency $>.5$ and <1, i.e., more than half but less than all).
2. A is F.
$\therefore$ C. A is G.

     1. *n* of *F* are *G.* (where *n* is a frequency <.5 and
        >0, i.e., less than half but more than none)
     2. *A* is *F.*
∴   *C. A* is not *G.*

These are also called *statistical syllogisms, proportional syllogisms, probabilistic syllogisms, myriokranic* (that is, thousand-headed) *syllogisms,* and *direct singular inferences.*

Frequency probability—the likelihood that a specific thing has a property, based strictly on the frequency with which all things of that sort have the property.

Frequency statement—a statement of the following form: *n* of *F* are *G.* The variable *n* stands for some frequency, or proportion, stated in ordinary language (as with "almost all") or as a decimal, a fraction, or a percentage. The predicate in the *F* position is usually termed the *population,* while the predicate in the *G* position is usually termed the *property.* A frequency statement states that with a certain frequency (*n*), a certain population (*F*) has a certain property (*G*). Also called a *simple statistical hypothesis.*

General explanation—an explanation that can apply to a wide range of observable outcomes. Newton's theories, for example, although applied in the text to Halley's comet, actually cover the motion of all objects at all times. General explanations are typical of science, though are not restricted to it.

Generality—possessed by a term that allows for degrees.

Genetic fallacy—a fallacy that evaluates a belief according to its source (that is, its genesis—thus, *genetic*) rather than according to the relevant evidence. The *ad hominem* fallacy and the fallacy of appealing to authority are examples.

Good reasoning—the sort of thinking most likely to result in your having good reasons and, thus, the sort of thinking most likely to give you knowledge.

Grab sampling—the process of including in your sample whatever members of the population happen to come your way. This is a failure of randomness.

If-then argument—one of a loosely defined group of deductive arguments that have an if-then statement as a premise. Also known as a *conditional argument* or *hypothetical syllogism.*

If-then dilemma—a valid dilemma that is constructed like any either-or dilemmas, except for an if-clause prefixed both to the either-or premise and to the conclusion. The most common form is as follows:

1. If T, then P or Q.
2. If P then R.
3. If Q then R.
∴ C. If T, then R.

If-then statement—a statement in the form of *If P then Q.* Also known as a *conditional.*

Imperative function—the function of directing others to action. An example of a sentence with this function is *Speak into the microphone.*

Implicit statements—statements that are not spoken or written in any form, but are relied on by the arguer as a part of the argument.

Indirect argument—an argument that shows a statement is false by showing that it leads to an absurd consequence. This is sometimes, alternatively, used to show that the negation of the statement is true (which amounts to the same thing as showing that the belief itself is false). Sometimes also called a *reductio ad absurdum argument* or, for short, *reductio.*

Inductive argument—an argument in which the premises are intended merely to count toward, or make probable, the conclusion. To determine whether the logic of an inductive argument is successful, a good rule of thumb is to ask these questions:

Do the premises count toward the conclusion?

> If the premises were true, would that make the
> conclusion probable?
Alternatively termed *probabilistic, ampliative,* or *nondemonstrative*
argument.

Inductive generalization—an argument that draws general conclusions
about an entire population from samples taken of members of the
population. Form is:
> 1. *n* of sampled *F* are *G*. (Where n is *any*
> frequency, including 0 and 1.)
∴   *C. n* (+ or - *m*) of *F* are *G*.

Inductive strength—the measure of an inductive argument's logical
success (contrast with deductive validity) based on how probable the
premises make the conclusion. To be logically strong an inductive
argument must satisfy both the correct form condition and the total
evidence condition. There is a continuum of logical strength,
ranging from *no support* to *very weak* to *fairly strong* to *very strong.*

Inference—movement from premises to conclusion. Also, sometimes
simply a synonym for *simple argument.*

Inference indicator—a term that indicates movement from premise to
conclusion. (Also called an *illative.*) Examples are *because,* which
introduces premises, and *therefore,* which introduces conclusions.

Inferential evidence—beliefs that are appealed to in support of another
belief (which is *inferred* from them).

Inferred analog—in an argument from analogy, the item in question,
about which the argument is drawing its conclusion.

Inferred similarity—in an argument from analogy, the property that the
inferred analog is alleged to have because the basic analog has it.

Intellectual honesty—wanting, above all, to know the truth about the
questions you care about.

Intellectual virtues—habits of thinking that are conducive to knowledge by making it more likely that the answers you arrive at are well reasoned.

Interrogative function—the function of asking a question. An example of a sentence with this function is *Are you now or have you ever been a member of the Communist party?*

Invalid—a deductive argument that is not logically successful. An argument is invalid if and only if it is possible for an argument with such a form to have true premises and a false conclusion.

Law of noncontradiction—no statement is both true and false. It follows from this that truth is objective and absolute—there cannot be any statement, for example, that is true for you but false for me.

Law of the excluded middle—every statement is either true or false. It follows from this that there is no middle ground between the true and the false.

Lexical ambiguity—semantic ambiguity in which the competing meanings are due to different definitions of a term (thus *lexical*, indicating that a lexicon, or dictionary, might define the term in more than one way).

Logic—the reasonableness conferred on an argument's conclusion by its premises. In an argument that is logically successful the conclusion *follows from* the premises—or, to put it differently, the premises *support* the conclusion. In deductive arguments, this is strictly a matter of the fit of the conclusion to the premises. In inductive arguments, it is also a matter of the fit of the conclusion to the total available evidence.

Logical argument—an argument in which the premises strongly support the conclusion, that is, the premises make it reasonable to believe the conclusion.

Logical constant—an expression that provides an argument with its logical form. Constants cannot vary without varying the form of the argument. Also called *connectives*.

Logical implication—those things that must be true if the statement is true; if they were not true, there would be no imaginable way in which the statement could be true. Logical implications are included within the literal meaning of the statement.

Main conclusion—the most important conclusion of a complex argument, the one that answers the question being asked in the broader conversation.

Margin of error—in the conclusion to an inductive generalization, the range of frequencies within which the property is stated to occur. Also called the *confidence interval*.

Misunderstood sample—when the method used for collecting information about the sample is not entirely reliable it results in a misunderstanding of the sample's properties, rendering the premise false. The more hidden the property (people's attitudes, for example, are easily hidden), the more likely the misunderstanding.

Motive-based fallacy—a fallacy that reflects a flaw in the motives that an argument tends to promote. Typically such a fallacy does result in a flaw in at least one of the four merits of an argument, but the location of the flaw in the argument itself may vary.

Name—an expression that identifies something to which, typically, properties are attributed. Names do not have to be proper names; for example, the expression *my teacher* in *My teacher is no slave to fashion* can serve as a name for our purposes. We are using the letters *A* through *E* as variables for names when describing logical form.

Noninferential evidence—things other than beliefs that are appealed to in support of a belief. This includes self-evidence and experiential evidence.

Observable outcome—what is explained in an explanatory argument; the observable outcome follows from the explanation and can in a certain way, at a certain time, and under certain conditions, be seen, heard, smelled, tasted, or touched. Also termed the *data*, the *prediction*, or the *facts*.

Part—a statement connected to another by *and*. Also known as *conjunct*.

Performative function—the function of doing, or performing, something by the very act of asserting it under the right circumstances. An example of a sentence with this function is *I promise to return the money on Tuesday*.

Predicate—an expression that identifies a property or attribute that can be ascribed to the thing named. We are using the letters *F* through *O* as variables for predicates when describing an argument's form.

Predicate logic—the branch of logic that deals with logical relationships among names and predicates. This is also sometimes called *quantifier logic* because these arguments include quantity terms like *all*.

Premise—any statement that is offered as a reason for belief in another statement. (Sometimes spelled *premiss* by the British.) We alternatively refer to premises as the *evidence, warrant, justification, basis, grounds*, or *rationale*. There must be at least one premise in an argument, but there is no upper limit.

Principle of charity—requires that you adopt the paraphrase that makes the arguer as reasonable as possible. This principle provides a way of aiming for the arguer's intentions when the context is unhelpful, and thus is subordinate to the principle of loyalty.

Principle of loyalty—requires that your clarification aim to remain true to the arguer's intent. Imagine that the arguer is looking over your shoulder.

Prior probability—the epistemic probability of a belief independent of (i.e., prior to) a specified piece of evidence. When considering, for example, the prior probability of something you heard, its prior probability is simply how probable it would be if you had not heard it.

Process of elimination—a valid form of either-or argument in which premises eliminate alternatives, while the conclusion includes all the alternatives that have not been eliminated by a premise. Examples include:

$$\begin{array}{ll} & \text{1. } P \text{ or } Q \\ & \text{2. Not } P \\ \therefore & C. \ Q \end{array}$$

$$\begin{array}{ll} & \text{1. } P \text{ or } Q \\ & \text{2. Not } Q \\ \therefore & C. \ P \end{array}$$

$$\begin{array}{ll} & \text{1. } P \text{ or } Q \text{ or } R \\ & \text{2. Not } P \\ \therefore & C. \ Q \text{ or } R \end{array}$$

$$\begin{array}{ll} & \text{1. } P \text{ or } Q \text{ or } R \\ & \text{2. Not } P \\ & \text{3. Not } Q \\ \therefore & C. \ R \end{array}$$

Also called *modus tollendo ponens,* which is Latin for "the method of denying in order to affirm."

Random selection—the process of selecting a sample such that every member of the population has had an equal opportunity to be included, so that exactly the relevant variations of the population might be proportionately represented.

Reasonable objector—someone who has approximately the same information you have, who exhibits the virtues of honesty, critical reflection, and inquiry, yet who disagrees with your evaluation. Imagine that this is your audience for every evaluation you write.

Reasoning—the attempt to answer a question by thinking about reasons.

Reasons—whatever you depend on in support of what you believe, regardless of whether you consider your belief to be knowledge or mere opinion. Words that mean more or less the same thing are the following: *premises, evidence, warrant, justification, basis, grounds,* and *rationale.*

Referential ambiguity—semantic ambiguity in which more than one thing might plausibly be picked out, or referred to, by a term.

Report indicator—shows that the argument is being reported by, but is not necessarily embraced by, the speaker or writer. *So-and-so argues that* is an example.

Rhetoric—principles of persuasive writing or speaking. Rhetoric can help or hurt the argument's clarity. It helps when it is used to make good arguments easy to accept on their own merits.

Secondary assumptions—when an if-then statement is asserted, these are assumptions made, often implicit because they are not in doubt, about other factors besides the if-clause that contribute to the truth of the then-clause. Also known as *auxiliary hypotheses.*

Self-evidence—evidence that comes from understanding the very meanings of the words themselves in a statement. Statements that are self-evidently true or false can be seen to be true or false largely by virtue of understanding the words of the statement. Philosophers sometimes refer to these statements as *analytic a priori* statements; they are also sometimes described as statements that are seen to be true or false *by definition.*

Self-selected sampling—when members of the population decide for themselves whether to be included in the sample. This is a failure of randomness.

Semantic ambiguity—a term that has more than one plausible meaning and it is not clear which is intended. Also called *equivocation*, since different things are being called (*...vocation*) by the same (*equi...*) name.

Sentential logic—the branch of logic that deals with logical relationships among entire statements (which are a kind of *sentence*). This is also sometimes called *propositional logic* because statements are sometimes also called *propositions*. We are using the letters *P* through *Z* as variables for statements when describing the form of an argument of sentential logic.

Shortcuts in reasoning—quick and practical ways of arriving at answers to your questions that do not involve organized arguments. More formally called judgmental heuristics. *Heuristic* is closely related to the word *eureka*, which is Greek for "I found it!" According to legend, Archimedes shouted "Eureka" as he ran naked through the streets of ancient Athens, having hit upon an important idea as he bathed.

Similarity shortcut—relying on quickly noticed resemblance between the familiar and the unfamiliar as a shortcut in reasoning. This can be helpful but is not always supported by the evidence. Also called the representativeness heuristic.

Simple argument—a series of statements in which at least one of the statements is offered as reason for belief in another.

Simplification—a valid deductive form, as follows:
   1. *P* and *Q*
∴   *C. P*

Singular affirming the antecedent—valid affirming the antecedent in which the if-then premise is universal and the conclusion is about a single instance that is encompassed by the universal term.

Singular categorical argument—a deductive argument, either valid or invalid, with a universal categorical statement as a premise, but with a conclusion about a single instance that is included in the universal category. For example, a valid form is:
   1. All *F* are *G*.
   2. A is *F*.
∴   *C.* A is *G*.

Singular denying the consequent—valid denying the consequent in which the if-then premise is universal and the conclusion is about a single instance that is encompassed by the universal term.

Singular explanation—an explanation that is designed to apply only to a single thing or event. Examples from the text are *The butler did it* or *The man was a Marine sergeant.*

Singular transitivity of implication—valid transitivity of implication in which the if-then premises are universal and the conclusion is about a single instance that is encompassed by the universal term.

Slanting—unjustifiably pointing a premise or conclusion towards the emotions rather than the reason of the audience.

Slippery slope fallacy—mistakenly concluding that because fuzzy borders can be harder to see, they are nonexistent.

Snowball sampling—the process of adding new members to the sample on the basis of their close relationship with those already included (thus gathering members in the same way that a snowball gathers snow as it rolls along). This is a failure of randomness.

Sound argument—an argument that both is logical and has true premises.

Sound but not shown—the evaluation to use under the *Soundness* subheading in a complex argument when one simple argument is sound, but a preceding simple argument, on which it depends, is unsound. Using this terminology reflects the fact that even though this simple argument happens to be sound, the arguer has failed to show it to be so, by virtue of having supported it with an unsound argument.

Specifying—paraphrasing in a way that narrows the range of possible things that an expression can mean, so as to increase the clarity of an argument.

Standard constant—when there are various ways of expressing the same constant, the one expression that we are adopting for use in the structuring of the argument. The alternative expressions are termed *stylistic variants* and are to be translated into the standard constant. For example, *if…then* is the standard constant, *assuming…then* is a stylistic variant of it.

Statement—a sentence that can be true or false. It functions to convey information. Its form, typically, includes a subject and a trait that is attributed to the subject.

Stipulative definition—a nonstandard definition for a term, decreed by a speaker or writer for some specific use.

Stratification—the construction of a random sample, for practical purposes, by identifying groups within the population that tend to be relatively uniform and including strata, or groups, of the sample in numbers that proportionally represent their membership in the entire population.

Straw man fallacy—uncharitably representing an argument or position in a way that makes it too easy to attack. This is a variety of the fallacy of missing the point (or *ignoratio elenchi*). This fallacy is so named because a straw man is a lightweight construction of one's own devising, much easier to knock down than a real man.

Streamlining—removal of nonessential features of the argument so that they will not get in the way of the evaluation process. It is one important aspect of the paraphrasing procedure.

Structuring—organizing your paraphrase of the argument so as to make its logical form as obvious as possible. This typically requires two procedures: translating stylistic variants into the standard constants, and matching the wording of statements, names, or predicates when they are expressed more than once in slightly different language.

Stylistic variant—when there are various ways of expressing the same constant, an expression that is to be translated into the standard constants. For example, *if...then* is the standard constant, *assuming...then* is a stylistic variant of it.

Subconclusion—in a complex argument, the conclusion of one simple argument that also serves as premise for the next simple argument.

Subjective probability—the degree of confidence you have that a given statement is true. It is entirely relative to the believer; there is no fact of the matter over and above the believer's level of confidence.

Syntactic ambiguity—the sort of ambiguity that occurs when the terms of an expression have more than one plausible grammatical relationship to one another, and when this results in lack of clarity about what the expression means. Also called *amphiboly*, from a Greek word for a special net that could be cast simultaneously on both sides of the boat, thereby catching twice as many fish—or meanings.

Total available evidence—all of the beliefs and experiences (i.e., the *total evidence*) that you as the evaluator personally have (i.e., that are *available* to you).

Total evidence condition—the logical requirement on any inductive argument that its conclusion fit appropriately with the total available evidence. Do not confuse this condition with the requirement of true premises. The total evidence condition bears on logic and is evaluated on the assumption that the premises are true; that is, this condition is to be evaluated as part of answering the question, "If the premises were true, would they make it reasonable for me to believe the conclusion?"

Transitivity of implication—a valid deductive form, as follows:
       1. If P then Q.
       2. If Q then R..
∴ C. If P then R..
It can have any number of if-then premises. It can also have a negative conclusion, as follows:
∴ C. If not R, then not P.

True statement—a statement that corresponds to the world.

Truth counterexample—a strategy for defending your judgment that a universal if-then premise is false by identifying a single instance in which the if clause is obviously true and the then-clause is obviously false.

Truth-values—evaluations, like *true* and *false,* which can be given of how well a statement fits with the world.

Universal statement—a premise with a term like *all, none, anything,* or *nothing.*

Unsound argument—an argument that has at least one false premise or is illogical (or both).

Use-mention distinction—the difference between the expression of a word to refer to the word itself—in which case the word is, strictly speaking, merely being *mentioned,* not used—and the other more ordinary expressions of the word, when it is being *used.* Confusion about this distinction can cause the sort of semantic ambiguity we have termed *referential ambiguity.*

Vagueness—the lack of a strictly defined boundary between what has a property and what does not have it.

Valid—a logically successful deductive argument. An argument is valid if and only if it is impossible for an argument with such a form to have true premises and a false conclusion.

Validity counterexample—a two step method for checking any argument for validity. The first step is to extract the form that the argument is depending on for logical success. The second step is to attempt to construct a new argument by appropriately substituting new sentences, predicates, or names in a way that produces obviously true premises and an obviously false conclusion.

Variable—a placeholder such as *P* and *Q* that indicates where the content can vary. It can appear only in a description of an argument's form, not in its clarification.

Vividness shortcut—relying on whatever information stands out most in your mind as a shortcut in reasoning. This can be helpful but is not always supported by the evidence. More formally called the *availability heuristic*.

Sample Answers to Odd Exercises

In many cases there is a range of right answers to an exercise; you and your instructor will probably be able to improve on many of the sample answers I provide. But there is an even wider range of wrong answers. These sample answers should give you a good idea of how to stay home on the right range. (When the exercise is to "make up" something and a sample answer is in the text, I have not provided an additional sample answer here.)

CHAPTER 1, SET (A)

1. Vividness. Probably failed, since plenty of cars with FOR SALE signs were probably there all along; because I now had a reason to be interested in them, I noticed them for the first time.
3. Similarity. The stars looked like frog eggs in the sky, so it seemed as though their origin could be that the moon laid them. Probably failed, of course, since the moon isn't a creature and doesn't have offspring.

CHAPTER 1, SET (C)

1. You don't seem to really want to know the truth about your bad grade—you just want to believe that it isn't your fault. So, self-interest is apparently your main motivation, and thus you aren't being intellectually honest. You aren't collecting relevant information that can bear on your conclusion (you ignore the professor's notes in the margins, for example), so you aren't showing evidence of the virtue of empirical inquiry. And you aren't paying attention to any arguments you may or may not have for blaming it on your professor, so you aren't being critically reflective.
3. Lysenko apparently wanted to support Marxist ideology and to remain in the good graces of the Communist leaders far more than he wanted to know the truth about whether wheat could inherit acquired characteristics. So he seems not to have been intellectually honest. Evidence from modern biological research was suppressed and changed—thus, he seems to have been lacking in empirical inquiry. And he didn't pay close attention to how good his own evidence was, so was deficient in critical reflection.

5. Arkadyevich seemed to be mainly concerned with adopting beliefs that fit with his personality and with those in his circle, not with knowing the truth. So he seems not to have been intellectually honest. He made no effort to collect additional information about these various beliefs, so lacked in empirical inquiry. And he didn't consider what his arguments were and whether they were any good, so was not critically reflective.

CHAPTER 2, SET (A)
1. The beach has a lot of sand.
3. The Communist party has fewer members than it used to.

CHAPTER 2, SET (B)
1. Form is interrogative. Function is interrogative (asking if you heard), can also be declarative (giving information that class was canceled). Could also be exclamatory if the circumstances are such that the speaker is astonished that you didn't hear.
3. Form is interrogative. Function is interrogative (asks if really expects it), can be declarative (saying that he is not credible) or exclamatory (showing surprise at his naïveté).
5. Form is declarative. Probably the only function is declarative.
7. Form is declarative. Probably the only function is declarative.
9. Form is imperative. Function is imperative (telling you to take the card along), can also be declarative (telling you that it is invaluable).

CHAPTER 2, SET (E)
1. From the fact that she lied it follows that she is not reliable. (It introduces the conclusion.)
3. We should close down the widget division. The justification is that nobody wants widgets anymore. (It introduces the premise.)
5. The party is over, so you should go home. (It introduces the conclusion.)

CHAPTER 2, SET (F)
1. So; introduces conclusion.
3. Shows that; introduces the conclusion.
5. For; introduces the premise. Jesus loves me, this I know, for the Bible tells me so.
7. Therefore; introduces the conclusion.

9. No indicator; not an argument.
11. Hence; introduces the conclusion.

CHAPTER 2, SET (G)

1. Conclusion: You aren't my real mother. No inference indicator.
3. Conclusion: It is a mirage. No inference indicator.
5. Conclusion: If the business moves to more services and processing, we'll move with it. Inference indicator: so, introduces the conclusion.
7. Conclusion: Eric Vallesteros has a life. No inference indicator.
9. Conclusion: I should turn my attention to finding the secret of happiness rather than the secret of the universe. Inference indicator: therefore, introduces the conclusion.

CHAPTER 2, SET (J)

1. Mere explanation. No reason is given to believe that anyone is going to push the button, for example.
3. Mere explanation. It is presented as an answer to a question about the cause of their falling down (so it isn't also offered as a reason to believe they fell down).

CHAPTER 2, SET (K)

1. Conclusion: You should be more generous with allowances.
3. Premise: The proof was the only copy of the stroy that existed.
5. Premise: The music of the Ramones is not notated. Premise: The music of Ives and Copland is notated.
7. Premise: Steinbrenner would not do anything wrong.

CHAPTER 2, SET (L)

1. Subconclusion: You were not born in the United States. Conclusion: You can never become President of the United States.
3. Subconclusion: You are a prime candidate for our graduate program. Conclusion: You should expect to have funding for your schooling next year.
5. Subconclusion: Twain does not take slavery seriously. Conclusion: Twain does not take black people seriously.
7. Subconclusion: The power of Marxism cannot be explained solely by his theories. Conclusion: The power of Marxism must therefore be located to a considerable degree in its religious impulse and its moral protest.

CHAPTER 2, SET (M)

1. First conclusion: By the fifth century A.D. literacy had worked its way into culture. Second conclusion: In the fifth century A.D. literacy was rare.

CHAPTER 2, SET (N)

1. Mere explanation.
3. Mere explanation.
5. Mere illustration.
7. Argument. Conclusion: Beavers react aggressively to the presence of a trespasser's scent mound.
9. Mere explanation (of why robots appeal to us, and why we prefer them to human slaves).
11. Mere illustration.

CHAPTER 3, SET (A)

1.
> 1. With her TV antenna the rural Texas woman could not even get Dallas.
> ∴ C. TV pictures could not come all the way from the moon.

3.
> 1. Personal relationships and subjective circumstances are very important in Japanese business dealings.
> ∴ C. Business agreements with Japanese businessmen must be accompanied by thorough discussions to ensure everyone really understands and agrees to each point.

CHAPTER 3, SET (B)

1. Logical implication. Conversational implication: I have some doubt about whether you intend to turn in your final paper.
3. Conversational implication. Logical implication: He would die if she left.
5. Conversational implication. Logical implication: The car is not worth the selling price.

CHAPTER 3, SET (C)

1. This student is not especially good at philosophy.
3. He is not the sort of friend you can depend on.

5. I don't have the phone number.
7. She did stay all night with the man in New York and Chicago.

CHAPTER 3, SET (D)

1. It seems to say that if you use their service you'll really be stuck. Presumably it really means that you'll never again go anywhere for repairs besides this service.
3. It's doubtful that ethical behavior in infants was improving, and likely that *mortality* is what was intended.
5. The store probably means to advertise that it is unrivaled *in convenience*, unrivaled inconvenience not being something that is likely to attract customers.
7. This description—which probably refers to logical people, not just men—is so extreme that it almost certainly isn't intended literally. There must be instances in which a logical man isn't self-righteous, and instances in which a reasonable man is wrong. It is more charitable to take this as saying that narrowly logical people tend to be self-righteous and insensitive to the human dimension, unlike more broadly reasonable people.

CHAPTER 3, SET (E)

1.
    1. The walking speed of dinosaurs averaged about 3 mph.
    2. Walking speed reflects an animal's metabolism
    3. Warm-blooded animals have a walking speed of about 3 mph.
∴   C. Dinosaurs were warm-blooded

3.
    1. If psychic power existed, then psychics would report that it is affected by distance.
    2. Psychics do not report that psychic power is affected by distance.
∴   C. Psychic power does not exist.

5.
    1. Two-thirds of the buildup CO_2 has taken place since 1940.
    2. Ocean temperature is the same as it was in 1940.
∴   C. Global warming forecasts are wrong.

CHAPTER 4, SET (A)
1. You should be careful.
3. You should take the way that is harder.
5. There is nothing wrong with whites raising their family apart from non-whites; whites have no responsibility to others.

CHAPTER 4, SET (B)
1. Although you are short on cash, I think you should buy your mother an answering machine, since you never get any credit for the times you call and she isn't in.
3. Because of all the cultural diversity, Louisiana is a great state to live in—despite the humidity.
5. Women are much more attuned to people's feelings, so, even though they tend to be encouraged to pursue other professions, they make better doctors than men.

CHAPTER 4, SET (C)
1. Discount: Stealing computer programs is illegal. Discount indicator: but.
3. Discount: Ours may be an age of reason—or at least high-tech reducibility. Discount indicator: but.
5. Discount: The United States remains the largest single market for telecommunications equipment, with approximately $15 billion in sales last year. Discount indicator: although.
7. Discount: Roger Sessions and Elliot Carter are composers of undoubted stature and Charles Ives is a most intriguing "original." Discount indicator: however.

CHAPTER 4, SET (D)
1. The stress level in the ground in Southern California is building back to the point where there will be another great earthquake.
3.
      1. Creationism is the only other explanation of origins besides evolution.
      2. Evolution is false.
∴   C. Creationism is true.
      1. The theory of evolution exists.
∴   C. It is permissible to teach evolution.

CHAPTER 4, SET (E)

1.

    1. This widget is unique.

∴   C. You should buy this widget.

3.

    1. You shouldn't burden authorities.

∴   C. You should let authorities make their decisions.

5.

    1. Humans are naturally social.

    2. It is better to socialize with friends than strangers.

∴   C. The happy person needs friends.

7. Rhetoric gets more followers than does reason.

CHAPTER 4, SET (F)

1.

    1. Republicans only want to enrich themselves.

    2. Republicans don't care about the underprivileged.

∴   C. You should not vote for Republicans.

3.

    1. A high rise would not fit the humane scale of the proposed site.

∴   C. A high rise should not be built on the proposed site.

5.

    1. Most people in England are speaking French.

∴   C. Most people in England shouldn't be speaking French.

7.

    1. Humans, especially physicians, should oppose the torture and death of any living thing.

    2. Antibiotics cause the torture and death of living bacteria.

∴   C. Antibiotics should be banned.

CHAPTER 4, SET (G)

1.

> 1. Almost all major scientific ideas arise independently and around the same time.
> ∴ C. Great scientists are embedded in their cultures.

3.

> 1. Jeffrey Potter's oral biography of Jackson Pollock is made up entirely of quotations.
> 2. Copyright laws do not cover quotations from other people.
> ∴ C. Jeffrey Potter's oral biography of Jackson Pollock is not protected by copyright laws.

5.

> 1. Intelligence professionals do not take chances due to compassion.
> ∴ 2. Philby alerted his fellow spies not out of compassion but to protect an important spy.
> ∴ C. There is a high-ranking spy in the West's foreign policy establishment.

7.

> 1. It is absurd to believe that the Son of God died.
> ∴ C. The Son of God died.
> 1. It is impossible that the Son of God was buried and rose again.
> ∴ C. The Son of God was buried and rose again.

CHAPTER 5, SET (A)

1. Work stoppage or a fish on the line (there are other possibilities too). I wasn't expecting a fish to take my bait.
3. Applauded or helped her out. The entire group applauded.

CHAPTER 5, SET (B)

1. *Time* magazine or our measure of the succession of events. *Time* magazine really confuses me sometimes.
3. Jack or Jack's father. Look—Jack is wearing sunglasses; if his father doesn't recognize him, Jack is going to be really upset.

CHAPTER 5, SET (C)

1. In biblical times, a man could have as many wives at the same time as he could afford. Elliptically ambiguous—unclear whether "at the same time" or "in succession" is omitted.

3. Except for a dog, a book is man's best friend. "Outside" is lexically ambiguous.

5. The period of our lives when heaven is all around us. "Lies about us" is lexically ambiguous.

7. You must speak aloud all your answers. "Oral" is referentially ambiguous—producing the use-mention confusion, since Gary thinks the attorney is referring to the word itself.

9. I would like to know her name. Elliptical ambiguity—presumably it isn't clear whether "to know" or "to take" is omitted.

CHAPTER 5, SET (D)

1.

    1. I'm required to write a term paper on the subject of the belly of a frog.

    2. There isn't much space on the surface of the belly of a frog.

∴   C. It will be difficult to satisfy the requirement to write a term paper on the subject of the belly of a frog.

3.

    1. Academics publish the results of their research or academics fail in their careers.

    [2. This academic has not published the results of his research.]

∴   C. This academic will die.

CHAPTER 5, SET (E)

1. Since 1985, forty-six percent of biology graduates and 40 percent of physical sciences graduates at the University have been women

3. University of Florida microbiologist Lonni Ingram holds the nation's five millionth patent, which is on how to convert trash to ethanol.

5. If you have any relevant information or prejudice in your minds, I must ask you to banish it.

7. I know that the King is English and that the Queen is English."

CHAPTER 5, SET (F)

1. "Raised" could range from having spent all my growing-up years there to having spent three or four of my most impressionable years there as a youth.
3. A "bull market" could have been inching its way up for a few weeks, or could have been increasing dramatically for years.
5. "Studied" can range from having focused all attention on the topic for days to having looked over the notes the night before while watching TV.

CHAPTER 5, SET (G)

1. Can be vague. A woman who is 5 feet 7 inches tall is somewhere around the border.
3. Can be vague. Someone who is moving quickly but not quite jogging can be on the border.
5. Can be vague. Ancient ancestors of homo sapiens who are of a different species but very close to homo sapiens in intelligence and appearance might be on the border.

CHAPTER 5, SET (H)

1.
    1. The store provides a free <u>pair of earrings</u>.
    2. I don't need a free <u>pair of ears.</u>
    ∴ C. I should not accept the store's offer.

3.
    1. If any student <u>steals a test,</u> that student will be expelled.
    2. All students are required to <u>submit to a test</u>.
    ∴ C. All students who do as required will be expelled.

5.
    1. Humans are life that <u>occupies space</u>.
    ∴ C. Humans are evidence that there is life <u>in outer space.</u>

7.
    1. All actions are motivated.
    ∴ 2. All actions are done because we <u>want, whether selfishly or not,</u> to do them.
    3. To do what you <u>selfishly want</u> is to be selfish.

∴   C. There could be no such thing as unselfish action.

CHAPTER 6, SET (A)
1. *P*: She could remember the phone number.
3. *P*: The band will sign with MCA. *Q*. The band will sign with Geffen Records.

CHAPTER 6, SET (B)
1. *F*: is a large state. *G*: has mountains.
3. *A*: the band. *F*: will sign with Geffen Records.

CHAPTER 6, SET (C)
1. Not *P*.
3. *P* or *Q*.

CHAPTER 6, SET (D)
1. All things that go up must come down.
3. Boston is a city with a rich history.
5. It is not the case that you will catch your plane.

CHAPTER 6, SET (E)
1.
     1. All great universities have excellent libraries.
     2. Oxford University is a great university.
∴   C. Oxford University has an excellent library.

3.
     1. Most who would go into the death hogan would be white men.
     [2. The horse thief went into the death hogan.]
∴   C. The horse thief was a white man.

5.
     1. If morality were simply conformity to the customs of one's group, then we could not justifiably criticize and improve our group's morals.
     2. We can justifiably criticize and improve our group's morals.
∴   C. Morality is not simply conformity to the customs of one's group.

CHAPTER 7, SET (A)

1. SOUNDNESS. The argument is unsound, since it is invalid.
3. SOUNDNESS. The argument is unsound, since premise 1 is certainly false.
5. SOUNDNESS. I can't decide about its soundness, since I can't decide about premise 2.

CHAPTER 7, SET (B)

1. a) All premises are almost certainly true and logic is successful.
   b) At least one premise is probably true (and no premise less than probably true) and logic is successful.
   c) A premise is almost certainly false or logic is unsuccessful or both.
   d) All premises are almost certainly true and logic is successful, but is an inference in a complex argument that comes after another inference that is not sound.
   e) Can't decide about at least one of the premises (and no premise comes out worse than can't decide) or can't decide about the logic of the argument (which would typically only happen with certain inductive arguments) or both.

CHAPTER 8, SET (A)

1. Doesn't commit the fallacy of missing the point, since the truth of all three of these claims is enough to establish that my team is better.
3. Commits the fallacy of missing the point, since the question remains whether democracy worked well in ancient Athens and, even if it did, whether the experience of ancient Athens applies to our own experience, and, even if it does, whether it compares favorably to communism.
5. Commits the fallacy of missing the point, since Stewart Granger has nothing to do with the point.

CHAPTER 8, SET (B)

1. Chevys have always been better than Fords because even GM's bottom-of-the line model is better than anything Henry Ford's company can produce.
3. Because the bull market is sure to continue, the stock market will keep going up.

CHAPTER 8, SET (C)

1. This is not an *ad hominem* fallacy. The claim depends upon the reliability of the two scientists, and the argument makes two points that directly aim to undermine their reliability.
3. Commits the *ad hominem* fallacy. The kind of car driven by the bill's sponsor might lead the crowd to dislike him, but presumably has nothing to do with the merits of the bill.

CHAPTER 8, SET (D)

1. There is nothing fallacious about this appeal to authority. Cousteau is a well-informed expert in this area, and his views on the subject are worth considering.
3. Probably a fallacious appeal to authority. Even though the mayor may well be telling the truth, the mayor has a conflict of interest and to encourage the reporter to take the mayor's word for it is to discourage good reasoning.

CHAPTER 8, SET (E)

1. This is legitimate, since feeling sorry for the children can be relevant to your doing something to help them.
3. This is legitimate, since your feeling about the hitchhiker can be relevant to whether you should pick him up.

CHAPTER 8, SET (F)

1. This is a fallacious appeal to consequences—wishful thinking is determining a belief about the way the world is.
3. This is a legitimate appeal to consequences, since the consequences are being brought to bear on what you should do.

CHAPTER 8, SET (G)

1. Fallacy of appealing to consequences, since wishful thinking is the only thing appealed to in order to encourage the belief in Santa Claus.
3. Fallacy of appealing to sympathy, since none of these considerations have anything to do with whether Kidd is really guilty, but simply try to take advantage of sympathetic feelings.
5. Fallacy of appealing to authority, since there is an explicit attempt to bring about submission to views of famous thinkers rather than to promote reflection about the question, in a case where the thinkers

were probably not in a position of special expertise (the issue vaguely defined as "human deterioration").

CHAPTER 9, SET (A)
1. Harleys sound better to me than any other bike on the road.
3. In 1997 the United States enjoyed a boom in the stock market.

CHAPTER 9, SET (B)
1. A pencil is an instrument for writing. Rivers flow downhill.
3. The North Pole is colder than the South Pole. We will someday put an astronaut on Mars.

CHAPTER 9, SET (C)
1. It could be that polls of the members of the state congress indicate that it has the support of only a small minority, thus making the epistemic probability low. You may, however, want it to pass so badly that you nevertheless believe that in the remaining few days the minority will be able to persuade the majority to change their votes—so, the subjective probability is high.
3. The epistemic probability for this might be quite low—suppose he has a reputation for fairness, he provided extensive explanations for how he arrived at the grade, and, on the other hand, you put very little effort into the paper. Still, the subjective probability is high if you firmly believe it—perhaps because you have trouble taking responsibility for your mistakes.
5. Perhaps the epistemic probability is on the fence—the evidence doesn't point clearly in either direction. But you've always dreamed of all the fun you would have playing ball with your son, and thus you believe it will be a boy.
7. Perhaps you've never been on empty before, so you have no evidence one way or the other regarding how accurate your gas gauge is. That makes the epistemic probability indeterminate. But, knowing that you're on a tight schedule and that you are a long way from the next town, you believe there's a lot of room under the empty line—which gives the belief a high subjective probability.

CHAPTER 9, SET (D)
1. Self-evidently true.
3. Neither.

5. Self-evidently true.
7. Self-evidently false.

CHAPTER 9, SET (E)

1. If I provide you with some token of affection that I'm not obligated to provide, then that counts as a gift. The voice mail I left wasn't obligatory, and it surely was a token of affection. So, I did too give you a birthday gift.
3. You're not going to arrest me, are you? It isn't stealing if the value is less then a dollar and if I intended to come back and pay for it later. This candy bar was only $.79. And I was going to come back later with the money, anyhow.

CHAPTER 9, SET (F)

1. Nobody else hears it—further, your doctor told you recently that you may be suffering from tinnitis (a hearing problem that produces a whistling sound).
3. Your mother has been dead for ten years. Your brother sees the same person and comments on her faint resemblance to your mother.
5. All your friends remember his saying that there would be no final exam when hell froze over, and the syllabus shows that the final exam counts for 100 percent of the grade in the class.
7. You are uncommonly afraid of spiders, often imagining that you feel one when it isn't there. Also, you're indoors, in a place where a spider is unlikely.

CHAPTER 9, SET (G)

1. The station making the announcement is presenting itself as the authority. The claim is that their interview will be definitive. It is less than reliable because scandals revolving around the president are seldom settled by interviews with the president (thus the prior probability is quite low); and the station is in the position to have self-interested motives in making the claim.
3. The National Golf Foundation is presenting itself as the authority. Its claim is that golf is booming and will continue to do so. Its job is to paint a rosy picture, so, without any other evidence pointing one way or the other, there is no way to tell whether it is just doing its job or providing reliable information.

69

5. Ricky Don White is presenting himself as having special access to information about the Kennedy assassination. His claim is that his father was with the CIA, participated in the assassination, and killed Tippet afterwards. In the absence of any other corroborating evidence, this has a status that is no different from the hundreds of other such claims that have been made. Since, in addition, White is trying to make money on the deal, his claim has little credibility.

CHAPTER 9, SET (H)

1. Add the following: It might be objected that there are even stronger forces in favor of government's doing more and more for the people, which would cost more and more money. Although there are those who do feel that way, research indicates that most people will not stand for much more of their own money going for those purposes.

3. Add the following: It might be objected that small towns have less crime, which is also a powerful enhancement to the quality of life. But lack of crime doesn't itself provide high quality of life—it just helps provide a framework for it. If there isn't anything to attach to the framework—which is what is provided by big-city cultural opportunities—then what good is the framework? Better to work at lowering or avoiding crime in the city.

CHAPTER 9, SET (I)

1. This is certainly true. Assume that it's false. This would mean that every male is married. But this is preposterous—it would mean that priests, widowers, and babies are married.

3. This is certainly true. Assume it is false. This would mean the richest people are the smartest people—thus, for example, the membership of Mensa would also constitute the roster of the wealthiest people. But there is no correlation between the two. Mensa members frequently don't have the interest, the ambition, the industriousness, or the people skills that can also help in creating wealth.

CHAPTER 10, SET (A)

1. Can't say.
3. Invalid.
5. Can't say.

CHAPTER 10, SET (B)
1.

    1. General Motors makes cars.

∴   C. Dogs are invertebrates.

3.

    1. If women in America hadn't wanted to vote before the 19th amendment was passed in 1920, then they would not have been allowed to vote before the 19th amendment was passed in 1920.

    2. Women in America did want to vote before the 19th amendment was passed in 1920.

∴   C. Women in America were allowed to vote before the 19th amendment was passed in 1920.

5.

    1. Venus is a planet in our solar system or it is always cold in the desert.

    2. Venus is a planet in our solar system.

∴   C. It is always cold in the desert.

CHAPTER 10, SET (C)
1.

    1. It is not the case that God does not exist.

∴   C. God exists.

    Valid by double negation.

3.

    1. Being married is good.

∴   C. Being married is good.

    Valid by repetition.

5.

    1. America is a country.

    2. America is free.

∴   C. America is a country and America is free.

    Valid by conjunction.

CHAPTER 10, SET (D)
1. (a) Valid by simplification. (b) Invalid. Commits the fallacy of division.

CHAPTER 10, SET (E)
1. .80 times .70 is .56, so the both-and statement is just slightly probably true.
3. .90 times .80 (since I must use the probability that Q is true *when I assume that P is true*) is .72, so it is somewhat probable that the both-and statement is true.

CHAPTER 11, SET (A)
1. If you were late, then your paycheck was docked. You were late. So your paycheck was docked.
3. If this is a tattoo, then it will resist soap and water. It does not resist soap and water. So, it is not a tattoo.

CHAPTER 11, SET (B)
1. If combustion occurs, then oxygen is present.
3. If the teacher consistently assigns a passage and requires the student to summarize it in the student's own words, then the student will not only learn to write a lot better but will also learn to analyze, evaluate, sort out, and synthesize information.
5. If you address kids in masses, then you are an entertainer.

CHAPTER 11, SET (C)
1.
    1. If a therapeutic intervention is available for AIDS or an infectious state puts others at risk of AIDS by casual contact, then universal mandatory screening for AIDS is justified.
    2. Therapeutic intervention is not available for AIDS and an infectious state does not put others at risk of AIDS by casual contact.
∴   C. Universal mandatory screening for AIDS is not justified.
    Invalid, fallacy of denying the antecedent.

3.
    1. If the North Koreans are smart, then they will move in the direction of reform.

    2.   The North Koreans are smart.

∴   [C. The North Koreans will move in the direction of reform.]
Valid, affirming the antecedent.

5.

    1.   If the fraternity is responsible, then the whole fraternity
system is responsible.

    2.   If the whole fraternity system is responsible, then our
educational institutions in general are responsible.

    3.   If our educational systems in general are responsible, then
our entire American society is responsible.

∴   [4. If the fraternity is responsible, then our entire American
society is responsible.]

    5. Our entire American society is not responsible.

∴   [C. The fraternity is not responsible.]
Argument to 4: valid, transitivity of implication
Argument to C: valid, denying the consequent.

CHAPTER 11, SET (D)
1.

    1.   If someone is in Birmingham, then that person is in
Alabama.

    2.   If someone is in Alabama, then that person is in America.

∴   C. If I am in Birmingham, then I am in America.
Valid, singular transitivity of implication.

3.

    1.   If anyone breaks a promise, then it is immoral.

    2.   An adulterous act breaks a promise.

∴   C. An adulterous act is immoral.
Valid, singular affirming the antecedent.

CHAPTER 11, SET (E)
1. Secondary assumptions. More people would listen to it. Those who
listen to it would increase their appreciation of it. Evaluation.
Probably true. These assumptions are probably true, as long as we are
assuming that the degree of increased appreciation is not enormous.

3. Secondary assumptions. You want to stay dry. You are going to work
tomorrow. You go outdoors when you go to work. Evaluation. Can't

decide if it is true, since in this context there is no clear way of saying what is referred to by terms like "you" and "tomorrow."

5. Secondary assumptions. I am at least of average height. I have athletic ability and interest that is at least average. If I had an excellent chance to make a lot of money by working very hard at improving my ability, I would. Evaluation. Probably true, since all the secondary assumptions are true.

7. Secondary assumptions. In the past, the entire market has tended to go in roughly the same direction as Microsoft. The trend of the past will continue in the future. Evaluation. I can't decide whether this if-then statement is true, since I haven't studied the trends carefully enough to know what the past trend has been, nor do I have any confidence in predicting the future trend.

9. Secondary assumptions. Ability to do twenty pushups is indicative of upper body strength. Upper body strength is a reliable indicator of being in good shape. Evaluation. This is, at best, a premise that can't be decided, and may well be false. The first secondary assumption is probably true, but the second one seems no better than fifty-fifty; I don't know the research, but it seems likely that there are a lot of people with a lot of upper body strength who are in bad shape and a lot of people in good shape who have average upper body strength.

CHAPTER 11, SET (F)

1. Certainly false. Geraldine Ferraro was a Democratic vice presidential candidate.
3. Certainly false. Newspapers reported that Dewey defeated Truman.
5. Certainly false. Beams of light go up and don't come down.

CHAPTER 11, SET (G)

1. I patched the hole myself, and we can all see the drops collecting on the beam in the living room. So the if-then statement is clearly false—though I have no idea where the new leak is.
3. There must be some explanation for the judge's decision that is yet to emerge. Everyone there believed that you were the best—you were the only performer they cheered, and they all booed when the winner was announced and it wasn't you. So, the if-then statement is obviously false.

CHAPTER 11, SET (H)
1.

    1. If it is acceptable for income taxes to be eliminated, then it is acceptable to allow the government to collapse.

    2. It is not acceptable to allow the government to collapse.

∴   C. It is not acceptable for income taxes to be eliminated.

The first premise is probably false, since the problem is probably not with the antecedent but with a false secondary assumption. One assumption is that there is no other source of income for the government to fund its necessary business. But there are other taxes, such as sales and property taxes, that it can impose.

CHAPTER 11, SET (I)
1.

    1. If evolution is true, then it took more time than the lifetime of the sun.

    2. It did not take more time than the lifetime of the sun.

∴   C. Evolution is not true.

Secondary assumption (which perhaps he should have questioned) is that Kelvin's thermodynamics are correct.

CHAPTER 11, SET (J)
1.

    [1. If anything is a high-tech innovation, it inevitably fragments community rather than enhancing it.]

    2. The Internet is a high-tech innovation.

∴   C. The Internet will fragment community rather than enhance it.

3.

    [1. If any innocent people are executed, then the death penalty should be abolished.]

    2. At least 23 innocent people have been executed.

∴   C. The death penalty should be abolished.

5.

    [1. If anything is of great worth and importance, then someone will try to steal it.]

    2. Nobody ever tried to steal a textbook.

∴   [C. Textbooks are not of great worth and importance.]

NOTE TO STUDENT: In the remainder of the sample answers there will be many examples of complete evaluations of arguments. Owing to space limitations, I have kept my evaluations fairly brief. Your instructor may want you to write a fuller evaluation than the sample answer I have provided (one that, for example, develops in more detail how you might respond to the reasonable objector over your shoulder). Consider these answers to be sketches of how you might start a fuller evaluation

CHAPTER 11, SET (K).

1.

1. If a rail line doesn't work in the San Francisco-Oakland area, then it will not work in Los Angeles.
2. A rail line doesn't work in the San Francisco-Oakland area.

∴   [C. A rail line will not work in Los Angeles.]

EVALUATION

TRUTH
Premise 1. The secondary assumptions—that the SF/Oakland area is more compact than LA, and that a rail line would work better in a more compact area—seem to be true; credence is also added to the premise by the fact that Gordon is apparently something of an expert, and there's no special reason to doubt him. So—not a lot to go on but somewhat probable that it's true.
Premise 2. On the one hand, Gordon is apparently an expert, and should know. On the other hand, I know people who use the rail line in the SF/Oakland area and think it works well. I can't decide.

LOGIC
Valid, affirming the antecedent

SOUNDNESS
Can't decide whether it is sound, since I can't decide about premise 2.

3.

1. If humans had definite rules of conduct by which they regulated all of their behavior, then they would be, in effect, machines.

2. Humans do not have definite rules of conduct by which they regulate all of their behavior.

∴ C. Humans are not, in effect, machines.

EVALUATION
TRUTH
Premise 1. Being charitable, I assume he is imagining that *all behavior* is governed by formulas (since the premise would be clearly false if it simply claimed that people who followed broad principles were machines). In that case, an important secondary assumption is that free will distinguishes humans from machines; another is that we would have no free will if all our behavior were formula driven. Both of these assumptions are very probably true, so I'd say the premise is probably true.
Premise 2. My experience of humans, including myself, is that most humans have principles they try to follow in some situations, but that these aren't strict rules and they don't cover nearly all of our behavior. So, it is almost certainly true.

LOGIC
Invalid, fallacy of denying the antecedent. Here's a validity counterexample:

1. If Santa Monica beach is covered with gravel, then it is unpaved.
2. Santa Monica beach is not covered with gravel.

∴ C. Santa Monica beach is not unpaved.

SOUNDNESS
Unsound due to invalidity.

5.

1. If U.S. citizenship has any value for someone out of the country, then the U.S. government should protect U.S. citizen Pjeter Ivezaj from imprisonment in Yugoslavia for his participation in peaceful demonstrations.
2. U.S. citizenship has value for someone out of the country.

∴ C. The U.S. government should protect U.S. citizen Pjeter Ivezaj from imprisonment in Yugoslavia for his participation in peaceful demonstrations.

EVALUATION
TRUTH
Premise 1. The charitable paraphrase adds that the value is for someone who is out of the country—otherwise, the premise would be clearly false (since there are certainly valuable aspects to U.S. citizenship for those who are in America). A secondary assumption here is that protection from false arrest is really the only significant value to citizens who are out of the country—that seems true. Another is that Ivejaz shouldn't have been arrested—on this matter we just don't have any reliable information (we know a little bit from his brother—who can't be counted on to be objective, and who can't be counted on to know the law). Can't decide.
Premise 2. Very probably true—I have little experience being out of the country, and little knowledge of the law, but my experience of American citizenship is that I would expect it to prove valuable even when out of the country.

LOGIC
Valid, affirming the antecedent.

SOUNDNESS
Can't decide on soundness, since I can't decide about premise 1.

7.

1. If God decided from all eternity for anyone who died of a disease that it should happen, then it would be wrong for humans to try to control disease.
2. God decided from all eternity for anyone who died of a disease that it should happen.
∴ C. It would be wrong for humans to try to control disease.

EVALUATION
TRUTH
Premise 1 seems to have as a secondary assumption that humans would be wrong to do anything that would interfere with a decision of God. But this seems certainly false. It is one thing for God to have a plan, quite another for humans to know exactly what it is. As long as humans don't know with certainty what

God's decisions are, then they should do what, by their lights, is the morally right thing. So, the premise is almost certainly false. Premise 2 is almost certainly false. If there is no God, then, of course, it is false. But even if there is a God, there is no good reason to think that this is the way he operates. He may know in advance of those who will die of disease, but this doesn't mean he will make it happen; he may know it because he may know which decisions people will make, which medicines people will discover, which efforts people will make to prevent disease, etc.

LOGIC
Valid, affirming the antecedent.

SOUNDNESS
Unsound, since both premises are false.

9.

1. If all have righteousness in their heart, then they will have beauty in their character.
2. If all have beauty in their character, then they will have harmony in their homes.
3. If all homes have harmony, then there will be order in the nation.
4. If all nations have order, then there will be peace in the world.
∴   [C. If all have righteousness in their heart, then there will be peace in the world.]

EVALUATION
TRUTH
Note: these premises are almost impossible to evaluate due to their vagueness. In each case, the secondary assumption is apparently something about the meaning of the term in the then-clause being somehow a part of what is meant by the term in the if-clause—a beautiful character, for example, just is a righteous heart. So, in the end, if the premises are true, they are self-evidently true (seen to be true by virtue of the meanings of the terms). But, due to the vagueness, I can't say that this is more

than probably the case. So, the premises are, at best, probably true.

LOGIC
Valid, transitivity of implication. (Note that, in order to be charitable, I had to paraphrase it in terms of "all" and "every" throughout; otherwise, it would not have been valid.)

SOUNDNESS
Probably sound.

11.

1. If children should be made free to reason through to their own answers about moral questions, then there are no answers to moral questions.
2. There are answers to many moral questions.
∴ C. Children should not be made free to reason through to their own answers about moral questions.

EVALUATION
TRUTH
Premise 1. The secondary assumption seems to be that by encouraging someone to reason through to an answer to a question, any answer the person arrives at is acceptable. This is certainly false. Someone can reason well or reason badly, and good reasoning is more likely to lead the person to the correct answer than bad reasoning. The premise is certainly false.
Premise 2. As long as it means "many moral questions," then it is almost certainly true. Does any reasonable person deny that there is an answer to whether the Nazis should have executed 6 million Jews? It may be objected that all of morality is just an expression of personal sentiment. But it is more than mere sentiment; to say "Abusing another person is wrong" is very different from saying "I hate the Green Bay Packers." It may include sentiment, but it makes a claim about moral truth. (This doesn't mean that it *is* true—but it does take care of the sentiment objection.) Or, it might be objected that all of morality is just an expression of the standards of one's own culture. But I can offer moral criticisms of my culture's standards—so my

moral criticisms are something different from—something over and above—my culture's standards.

LOGIC
Valid, denying the antecedent.

SOUNDNESS
Unsound, due to certainly false first premise.

CHAPTER 12, SET (A)

1. Mondale would have been a good president or Rockefeller would have been a good president.
3. A virus that later immobilizes the immune system cannot exist in a person's body for several years or a virus that later immobilizes the immune system causes serious ill effects.

CHAPTER 12, SET (B)

1.

    1. This is the best bunch of graduate students we've produced or I've lost my mind.
    [2. I have not lost my mind.]
∴   C. This is the best bunch of graduate students we've produced

3.

    1. A man gets bushwhacked for love or a man gets bushwhacked for money.
    2. The priest did not get bushwhacked for money.
∴   C. This priest got bushwhacked for love.

5.

    [1. The power of Marxism can be explained by Marx's theories or the power of Marxism can be explained by its religious impulse and moral protest.]
    2. The power of Marxism cannot be explained by Marx's theories.
∴   C. The power of Marxism can be explained by its religious impulse and moral protest.

CHAPTER 12, SET (C)

1. Therefore, George Strait will perform in town in April or Reba McIntyre will perform in town in April.
3. Therefore, we lost everything.
5. Therefore, the championship was won by the Lakers.

CHAPTER 12, SET (D)

1.

      1. You should major in something like business or you are committed to studying ideas for the sake of studying ideas.

      2. You are not committed to studying ideas for the sake of studying ideas.

∴   C. You should major in something like business.

      Valid, process of elimination.

3.

      1. Smith will teach the course or Jones will teach the course.

      2. Smith will not teach the course.

∴   C. Jones will teach the course.

      Valid, process of elimination.

CHAPTER 12, SET (E)

1. Add .30 and .05, then subtract .01, for .34. It is probably false.
3. Add .80 and .10, then subtract .00, for .90. It is very probably true.

CHAPTER 12, SET (F)

1.

      [1. Every person worries a lot or that person fails to worry enough.]

      2. If the person worries a lot, then the person is unhappy.

      3. If the person fails to worry enough, then the person is unhappy.

∴   [C. Every person is unhappy.]

EVALUATION

TRUTH

Premise 1. Certainly false. There are definitely people who do not worry a lot but who do worry enough (so they are counterexamples to this premise). Enough worrying is not necessarily a lot of worrying.

Premise 2. Almost certainly true. Smullyan's secondary assumption, as he says, is that worry tends to cause unhappiness, and this is consistent with my experience.

Premise 3. A secondary assumption here is that worry is necessary for taking precautions in order to ward off catastrophes. This is clearly false. You can take precautions without worrying—perhaps you just take precautions because you think it's a good idea, you take pleasure in taking precautions, etc. So the premise is almost certainly false.

LOGIC
Valid, correct form for either-or dilemma

SOUNDNESS
Unsound, due to two premises—1 and 3--that are certainly false.

3.

[1. Tarkanian keeps losing or Tarkanian quits]
2. If Tarkanian keeps losing, then Tarkanian suffers severe stress.
3. If Tarkanian quits, then Tarkanian suffers severe stress.
∴ [C. Tarkanian suffers severe stress.]

EVALUATION
TRUTH
Premise 1. I'm not sure whether Tarkanian kept losing—I have the vague impression that he usually won; but, if the sportswriter can be trusted (and we have no reason to mistrust him), he didn't quit. So, the first alternative is no better than .40 or so and the second is no better than .10. We add these (no chance that they are both true, so no subtraction is necessary) and get .50, so it seems that's there's no way to decide whether the premise is true.

Premises 2 and 3. Somewhat probable that they are true (note that I have charitably paraphrased "goes nuts" as "suffers severe stress"), given that there is no good reason to doubt the sources here, and it is a common condition for intensely competitive people.

LOGIC
Valid, correct form for either-or dilemma

SOUNDNESS
Can't decide whether it is sound, due to inability to decide about premise 1.

5.

[1. The fellow believes it when he says there is no distinction between virtue and vice or the fellow does not believe it when he says there is no distinction between virtue and vice.]

2. If the fellow believes it when he says there is no distinction between virtue and vice, then the fellow is not to be trusted.

3. If the fellow does not believe it when he says there is no distinction between virtue and vice, then the fellow is not to be trusted.

∴   [C. The fellow is not to be trusted.]

EVALUATION
TRUTH
Premise 1. This is almost certainly true—it is an instance of the law of the excluded middle (and there is no reason to think that it is one of the rare undecidable cases, such as, say, a case that is exactly on the borderline).
Premise 2. The secondary assumption here is that failure to believe in ethical absolutes will lead to behavior that society considers immoral. This is not compelling, however—such a person might well act in socially acceptable ways simply because the person is thoroughly socialized, or just prefers to get along smoothly in society. The assumption is probably false, as is the premise.
Premise 3. The secondary assumption here is that someone who does not tell the truth in one instance cannot, in general, be trusted. But many, many people lie in small ways yet at the same time can in general be trusted. If this fellow is lying, then he is pretending to have a philosophical belief he doesn't have—he is in effect, posturing. This may show a character defect, but doesn't seem to make it especially likely that he is in general

untrustworthy. So the assumption—and the premise—are probably false.

LOGIC
Valid, correct form for either-or dilemma

SOUNDNESS
Probably unsound, due to probable falsity of premises 2 and 3.

CHAPTER 12, SET (G)

1.
    1. If Dave Wilson gets a job next summer, then Dave Wilson will get a better car or Dave Wilson will move into a nicer apartment.
    2. If Dave Wilson gets a better car, then the money Dave Wilson earns will be gone.
    3. If Dave Wilson moves into a nicer apartment, then the money Dave Wilson earns will be gone.

∴ C. If Dave Wilson gets a job next summer, then the money Dave Wilson earns will be gone.

EVALUATION
TRUTH
Premise 1. One secondary assumption seems to be that my current job would not be expected to continue through the summer—thus, that my getting a summer job would enhance my anticipated financial condition. This is false—I already have a job year-round. So, the premise is almost certainly false.
Premises 2 and 3. These premises fail for the same reason as premise 1. A secondary assumption in each case is that my current job doesn't continue through the summer, and that I would be earning money from a summer job and then be spending about the same amount on a lifestyle enhancement. But the assumption is false, since my job does continue through the summer, and working in the summer wouldn't enhance my anticipated financial condition. [Note: many students may find these three premises true.]

LOGIC
Valid, correct form for if-then dilemma.

SOUNDNESS
Unsound, due to false premises.

3.

[1. If anyone wishes to get enlightened, then that person wishes
to be enlightened for self-improvement or that person wishes
to get enlightened in order to spread it to others.]
2. If anyone wishes to get enlightened for self-improvement,
then that person will be accused of selfishness.
3. If anyone wishes to get enlightened in order to spread it to
others, then that person will be accused of selfishness.
∴ [C. If anyone wishes to get enlightened, then that person will be
accused of vanity.]

EVALUATION
TRUTH
Premise 1. The secondary assumption is that there are only two
possible motivations for seeking enlightenment—helping oneself
and helping others. But this is certainly false—one might be
motivated by, say, the desire to please God or by simple
fascination with the goal regardless of whether anybody is
helped by it or not.
Premises 2 and 3. One key secondary assumption to both of
these premises is that all of us have cynics as friends—that is, all
of us have people as friends who would try to find the most
distasteful motives in whatever we do. This is certainly false—
some of us do, but others make a point of avoiding having such
people as friends. The only other thing that would make these
premises true is that all of us have stupid people as friends—
people who would confuse honest self-improvement with vanity
and honest altruism with self-aggrandizement. Again, some of
us do, but people this stupid are even rarer than cynics.

LOGIC
Valid, correct form for if-then dilemma.

SOUNDNESS
Unsound, due to falsity of all the premises.

CHAPTER 12, SET (H)
1.

    1. If anyone has an income of under $100,000 per year, then that person is not eligible.

    [2. You have an income of under $100,000 per year.]

∴   C. You are not eligible.

    Valid, singular affirming the antecedent.

3.

    1. If he cooks, then the food is delectable.

    2. He will cook tonight.

∴   C. The food tonight will be delectable.

    Valid, singular affirming the antecedent.

5.

    1. If anyone has a lean and hungry look, then that person is dangerous.

    2. Cassius has a lean and hungry look.

∴   [C. Cassius is dangerous.]

    Valid, singular affirming the antecedent.

CHAPTER 13, SET (A)
1.

    1. .90 of the time when a car's engine has steam coming out of it the car needs new hoses.

    [2. This car's engine has steam coming out of it.]

∴   C. This car needs new hoses.

    Correct form for frequency argument.

3.

    1. Less than .50 of the times when tackle is snagged on the lake bottom it comes loose.

    2. This is a time when tackle is snagged on the lake bottom.

∴   C. This is a time when it will not come loose.

    Correct form for frequency argument.

5.

      1. Most French painters late in the 19th century were impressionists.

      2. Seurat was an impressionist.

∴   C. Suerat was a late 19th century French painter.

Incorrect form for a frequency argument. Second premise must take the form *A is F*, but this one has the form *A is G*.

CHAPTER 13, SET (B)

1. Strong.
3. Very weak.
5. Fairly strong.

CHAPTER 13, SET (C)

1. No support. Even though the frequency in premise 1 is high, the frequency with which there is a need for new hoses when an engine *with new hoses* has steam coming out of it is very low—surely below half.

3. Very weak. This background evidence, of course, does not undermine the argument. But the argument itself cannot be stronger than the frequency it offers—and the frequency is merely "less than half." Clearly, you have better reasons for accepting the conclusion than those offered by this argument.

5. Fairly strong. This background evidence (as with exercise 3) gives better reason to believe the conclusion than does the argument. It doesn't undermine the argument, so it is as strong as is indicated by the .90 frequency.

CHAPTER 13, SET (D)

1.

      1. Most of what Peter Jennings says on the evening news about world news is true.

      2. That America has struck at terrorist bases in the Middle East is something that Peter Jennings says on the evening news.

∴   C. That America has struck at terrorist bases in the Middle East is true.

EVALUATION
TRUTH
Premise 1. This is almost certainly true. Jennings is a reliable reporter with a large news gathering organization behind him, all with a strong interest in maintaining a reputation for reliability. Premise 2. I can't decide—I have no way of evaluating this, since the passage says nothing about who is claiming this, when it is, etc.

LOGIC
Moderately strong frequency argument; it has correct form and no undermining evidence, but moderate strength is all we can assign it when the frequency is "most."

SOUNDNESS
Can't decide whether it is sound, since I can't decide whether premise 2 is true.

3.

1. Most of what the scholar's informant says is true.
2. The scholar's informant says that the person met by the scholar is dead.
∴ C. The person met by the scholar is dead.

EVALUATION
TRUTH
Premise 1 and 2. Can't decide. There is no way to judge these premises; there is no context to tell us who is being referred to, so there's no way to determine which background evidence to check.

LOGIC
No support. Correct form and moderately high frequency, but the background evidence—that the person is standing, alive, in front of the scholar—completely undercuts the report from the scholar's informant.

SOUNDNESS
Unsound, since the logic provides no support.

5.
1. Most of De Branges's claims to have proved an important theorem are false.
2. De Branges's claim to have proved the Bierbach conjecture is one of De Branges's claims to have proved an important theorem.
∴ C. De Branges's claim to have proved the Bierbach conjecture is false.

EVALUATION
TRUTH
Premise 1. Probably true, given that *Science News* is generally reliable, and one would expect a Duren, the University of Michigan mathematician, also to be reliable on this sort of report.
Premise 2. Probably true, given that *Science News* is generally reliable and there is no reason to doubt it in this case.

LOGIC
Moderately strong frequency argument, given that it has correct form and says "most," and that's the only information available to us (since we're assuming we don't have the extra information that the proof apparently succeeded).

SOUNDNESS
Probably moderately sound, since the premises are probably true and the logic is moderately strong.

CHAPTER 14, SET (A)
1. "Had" is the stylistic variant. Every sampled piece of pie at the Country Kitchen was delicious.
3. "Documented" is the stylistic variant. No sampled behavior of a healthy wolf is an attack by a healthy wolf on a human.
5. "X-rayed" is the stylistic variant. 60 percent of the sampled ex-football players have spinal damage.

CHAPTER 14, SET (C)
1. Almost every piece of pie at the Country Kitchen is delicious.

3. Almost no behavior of a healthy wolf is an attack by a healthy wolf on a human.
5. 60 percent (+/- 5 percent) of ex-football players have spinal damage.

CHAPTER 14, SET (D)

1.

    1. All sampled 13-ounce cans of Folger's coffee at this 7-Eleven cost $3.99.

∴   C. All 13-ounce cans of Folger's coffee at this 7-Eleven cost $3.99.

Property is "costs $3.99." It is probably an all-or-none property.

3.

    1. Most sampled opportunities to show intelligence do not show intelligence.

∴   C. Most opportunities to show intelligence do not show intelligence.

Property is "shows intelligence." It is not an all-or-none property; someone who shows intelligence in conversation, for example, may not show it in long division.

5.

    1. All sample people from Syracuse are of Norwegian descent.

∴   C. Most people from Syracuse are of Norwegian descent.

Property is "being of Norwegian descent." In these circumstances it is not an all-or-none property—you would expect diverse backgrounds among the population of a town like Syracuse.

CHAPTER 14, SET (E)

1. 50 percent (+/- 30 percent) of owners of 1999 Acuras are pleased with their cars.
3. 7 percent (+/- 10 percent) of the days in Atlanta are days with unhealthful levels of ozone in the air.
5. 48.3 percent (+/- 3 percent) of Texas adults believe the state sport should be rodeo.
7. 18 percent (+/- 4 percent) of Manhattan's streetlights are out of order.

CHAPTER 14, SET (F)

1. 27 percent of the sampled voters favor the third-party candidate, so 27 percent (+/- 4 percent) of the voters favor the third-party candidate. (Assume the sample includes 500 that are randomly selected.)
3. All dogs are mammals, Lassie is a dog, and so Lassie is a mammal.
5. If anybody asks you for a handout, then you should not give the person any money. The cashier did not ask you for a handout. So, you should not give her any money.

CHAPTER 14, SET (G)

1. Population: owners of 1999 Acuras. Property: being pleased with their car. Relevant variations: whether the car is used for business or pleasure; and whether this is the first luxury car owned by the person. Irrelevant variation: whether their names began with a letter in the first or last half of the alphabet.
3. Population: days in Atlanta. Property: having unhealthful levels of ozone in the air. Relevant variations: time of the year; kind of weather. Irrelevant variation: whether the mayor was in town that day.
5. Population: Texas adults. Property: believing the state sport should be rodeo. Relevant variations: gender, whether they live in the city or in the country. Irrelevant variation: whether phone number ends in odd number.
7. Population: Manhattan's streetlights. Property: being out of order. Relevant variations: whether in a good or bad part of town, whether in front of a police station or not. Irrelevant variation: what color the lamppost is painted.

CHAPTER 14, SET (H)

1.

1. About 2/3 of the sampled students at the community college doubted the practical value of their education.

∴ C. The majority of the students at the community college doubted the practical value of their education.

Sample is not large enough. For a random sample of thirty, the margin of error must be roughly 25 percent (extrapolating from the table on margins of error). That means that the margin of error would go as low as around 40 percent—but the conclusion calls for a majority. Also, it is not randomly selected. The sample is strictly from one English class. It probably does not include relevant variations—it may have a disproportionately large number of English majors, for example, who know that their degrees are not of great practical value.

3.

    1. 60 percent of the sampled drugs manufactured in one month are impure.

∴   C. Over half of the drugs manufactured in that month are impure.

Sample size is probably large enough—there is no way to be sure, since we aren't told, but it would be in the company's own interest to have a reliable quality control procedure, so, chances are they do. The sample is not randomly selected, however, since the sampling process itself introduces a relevant variation (the microscopic chemical residue from the cleaning) not found in the population.

5.

    1. All sampled young people are dressed in blue denim.

∴   C. Almost all young people dress in blue denim

Sample is too small. No reason to think this property is all-or-none, and even if the sample were random the margin of error would have to be in the neighborhood of 15 percent. But the sample is not random; it is a single "art-colony" village, which probably attracts a certain sort of resident.

7.

    1. 62 percent of sampled American adults favor allowing students and parents to choose which public schools in their community the students attend.

∴   [C. 62 percent (+/- 3 percent) of American adults favor allowing students and parents to choose which public schools in their community the students attend.]

Sample of 1,500 is plenty large enough, given the margin of error of 3 percent. It is probably randomly selected, since it is done by the professionals at Gallup and there is no reason to be suspicious of the result.

CHAPTER 14, SET (I)
1.

> 1. About 20 percent of the sampled voters favor George Wallace.

∴   C. About 20 percent of the voters favor George Wallace.

Premise 1 is almost certainly false. It is likely that the sample was randomly selected (reputable organizations did it); but it is easy to see, in retrospect, that many people would have been embarrassed to admit to a pollster that they favored someone with a racist reputation—even though they would not have minded casting a vote for him in the privacy of the booth. So, it's probably true that 20 percent of them said they favored Wallace, but not that 20 percent of them actually favored Wallace.

3.

> 1. About 95 percent of sampled customers of a fitness club looked better after two months in the program.

∴   C. About 95 percent of customers of a fitness club looked better after two months in the program.

Premise 1 is probably false. The subjects *believed* the customers looked better, but the only thing that is pretty clearly true is that the *photos* looked better.

NOTE TO STUDENT: In many of the sample evaluations that follow, the judgment "can't decide" turns up frequently. Don't be lulled into thinking that you should rely heavily upon "can't decide" in other cases as well. It occurs so often here because in many of the passages there is very little background information provided—sometimes no information about the source of the data and no information about the sampling procedure. In inductive generalizations, this sort of information can be crucial in being able to decide.

CHAPTER 14, SET (J)
1.

> 1. 95 percent of sampled golden retriever owners considered golden retrievers to be well behaved with children.

∴   2. About 95 percent of golden retriever owners consider golden retrievers to be well behaved with children.

    3. I will be a golden retriever owner.

∴   C. I will consider my golden retriever to be well behaved with children.

EVALUATION OF ARGUMENT TO 2
TRUTH
Premise 1 is undecidable. It could well be true—but I have no information about the source of this information, and thus reserve judgment.

LOGIC
This is also undecidable. A sample of 500, if randomly selected, calls for a margin of error of at least 4 percent, and this is consistent with the phrase "about 95 percent." But there is no way of knowing whether it is randomly selected.

SOUNDNESS
Can't decide whether it is sound, since can't decide about either the premise or the logic.

EVALUATION OF ARGUMENT TO C
TRUTH
I can't decide about premise 2. I wouldn't be surprised if it were true, since golden retrievers, in my experience, do have a good reputation for their gentleness with children, but it may be that, say, only 80 percent of the owners find them to have this quality.

LOGIC
Valid, singular categorical argument.

SOUNDNESS
Can't decide about soundness, since can't decide on premise 2.

CHAPTER 14, SET (K)
1.

    1. Most sampled teenage girls aspire to professional occupations.

∴   C. Most teenage girls aspire to professional occupations.

EVALUATION
TRUTH
Premise 1 is a statement I can't decide about, since there's no information about how the sampling was done and the claim is somewhat surprising--given the long history of culture-induced female preferences for other sorts of occupations, one would still expect a random sample to generate more boys than girls who aspire to professional jobs. Without any information about the way the sampling was done, it's best to reserve judgment.

LOGIC
Can't decide on the strength of the inductive generalization. Correct form, and given the vagueness of the conclusion, the sample seems large enough. But I can't decide whether it is randomly selected. It's possible to assemble a group of Illinois teenagers who represent all teenagers, I suppose, but there is no way to know whether, for example, it was self-selected or faulty in some other way.

SOUNDNESS
Can't decide if it's sound, since both premises and logic are undecidable due to poor information.

3.
    1. All sampled people who watched the Bugs Bunny/Road Runner show as kids without any of the violence cut weren't harmed by it.
∴   [C. Almost all people who watched the Bugs Bunny/Road Runner show as kids without any of the violence cut weren't harmed by it.

EVALUATION
TRUTH
Premise 1 can't be decided. We don't know anything about the writer, and recognize that it would be very difficult for someone to judge about himself or about someone else whether such TV violence did any harm.

LOGIC

Extremely weak logic in the inductive generalization. Correct form, but being harmed by TV violence is not an all-or-none sort of property, so a sample of one is useless.

SOUNDNESS

Unsound, due to weak logic.

5.

    1. 51 percent of the sampled American consumers feel guilty when buying non-American made products.

∴   C. 51 percent (+/- 2 percent) of the American consumers feel guilty when buying non-American made products.

EVALUATION

TRUTH

Premise 1 is probably true. The research company is reputable, as is the newspaper reporting the results, and the result has a reasonably high prior probability, so it is unlikely that their results are being misstated.

LOGIC

Fairly strong inductive generalization. Correct form. The sample is large enough for a 2 percent margin of error, and, although we aren't told about the selection process, again, the company knows how to do random samples, and the results aren't surprising, so it is probably randomly selected.

SOUNDNESS

Probably fairly sound.

CHAPTER 15, SET (A)

1. Basic analog: marriage. Inferred analog: employer-employee relationship. Basic similarity: that it is an important relationship. Inferred similarity: that counseling should be sought when there are difficulties.

    1. Marriage is an important relationship and the participants in a marriage should seek counseling when there are difficulties.

       [2. The employer-employee relationship is an important
         relationship.]

∴   C. The participants in an employer-employee relationship
         should seek counseling when there are difficulties.

3. Basic analog: streetcars, buses, subways, and trains. Inferred analog: elevators. Basic similarity: it is a means of transportation. Inferred similarity: men need not remove their hats when women are present.
      1.   Streetcars, buses, subways, and trains are means of transportation and men need not remove their hats in streetcars, buses, subways, and trains when women are present.
      2.   Elevators are means of transportation.

∴   C.   Men need not remove their hats in elevators when women are present .

5. Basic analog: a college junior who receives a lucrative job offer as a journalist. Inferred analog: a college junior who receives a lucrative job offer as a professional athlete. Basic similarity: that the student is getting a good opportunity in the student's chosen career. Inferred similarity: that the student should accept the offer.
      1.   A college junior who receives a lucrative job offer as a journalist is getting a good opportunity in the student's chosen career, and should accept the offer.
      2.   A college junior who receives a lucrative job offer as a professional athlete is getting a good opportunity in the student's chosen career.

∴   C.   A college junior who receives a lucrative job offer as a professional athlete should accept it.

CHAPTER 15, SET (B)

1. The basic similarity (that something is an important relationship) is relevant to the inferred similarity (that outside counseling should be sought when there are difficulties), since the importance of a relationship should certainly count in favor of any measures that might serve to improve it.
3. The basic similarity (that something is a means of transportation) may be somewhat relevant to the inferred similarity (that men need not remove their hats there when women are present), but it seems limited. Should men leave their hats on in restaurants on ocean

liners? Probably not. On escalators? Probably so. Other factors seem more likely to be far more relevant than whether something is a means of transportation.

5. The basic similarity (getting a good opportunity in the student's chosen career) is definitely relevant to the inferred similarity (that the student should accept the offer).

CHAPTER 15, SET (C)

1. (i) An irrelevant dissimilarity is that marriage involves people of the opposite sex, while employer-employee relationships are often of the same sex. This doesn't seem to count against whether outside counseling is a good idea. (Homosexuals who are not married are not bad candidates for outside counseling on the grounds that they are of the same sex.) (ii) A relevant dissimilarity is that marriage is essentially a social and interpersonal relationship while the employer-employee relationship is essentially a work—and thus performance-based—relationship. The goal is good performance, not a happy relationship. So if the difficulties are performance related, then the under-performer should be disciplined or fired. (iii) The argument fails the second part of the total evidence condition for analogical arguments, and is logically very weak.

3. (i) An irrelevant dissimilarity is that an elevator moves vertically while the others move horizontally. (When a train goes up a very steep mountain—getting closer to verticality—the men don't start thinking that perhaps they should put their hats back on in the presence of the women.) (ii). A relevant dissimilarity is that elevators are usually already indoors (no need to quickly put it back on again when you exit the means of transportation, as with buses and the like). Whatever rule applies to the use of stairs and escalators, it seems, should apply to elevators, and they seem to vary with whether they are indoors or out. (iii) So, the argument is very weak, since the similarity is only weakly relevant and there is a relevant dissimilarity.

5. (i) An irrelevant dissimilarity is that athletes usually handle a ball and journalists don't. (ii) A relevant dissimilarity is that the athlete's career is in an area that doesn't require the intellectual maturity provided by college, while the journalist's does. This means that the student who receives the journalism offer has probably already gotten a lot of intellectual value out of college, and will probably continue to grow intellectually in the career. The athlete may be more likely to

have a defect in this area—thus may benefit more, as a person (though not from a career point of view) from completing college than the journalist. (iii) It still seems to be a somewhat strong argument, since young people should be allowed to decide whether that is a cost they are willing to pay for the benefit of going on with their career.

CHAPTER 15, SET (D)

1.

       1. *Psycho* is a Hitchcock movie and is scary.

       2. *The Birds* is a Hitchcock movie.

∴   C. *The Birds* is scary.

(Note: this *could* also be clarified as a complex argument, with an inductive generalization from the one sampled Hitchcock movie to a conclusion about most Hitchcock movies, then a frequency argument from most Hitchcock movies to *The Birds*.)

    EVALUATION

    TRUTH

    Premise 1 is certainly true, based on my own experience (and what I know of the experience of many others). There is no reasonable objection.

    Premise 2 is certainly true, again, based on my own experience; there is no reasonable objection.

    LOGIC

    Fairly strong analogical argument. Correct form. Being a Hitchcock movie does make it likely that it's scary (at least in the sense of being very suspenseful), and there isn't any especially relevant dissimilarity between *The Birds* and *Psycho*.

    SOUNDNESS

    Fairly sound, since the logic is fairly strong.

3.

       1. J. Edgar Hoover did not advise people he was investigating that they were under investigation, and Hoover's behavior was appropriate.

       2. The university administration did not advise people they were investigating that they were under investigation.

∴   C. The university administration's behavior was appropriate.

EVALUATION
TRUTH
Premise 1 is highly controversial. It is true that Hoover didn't advise people that the FBI was investigating them, but in many cases it has been argued that the FBI violated their rights in this way. In certain cases, of course, investigation is necessary and telling someone about it would ruin the investigation. But Hoover crossed that line too often. It is probably false.
Premise 2 is, I presume true, since it seems to be the background assumption to the interview, and those who could deny it are not doing so.

LOGIC
Extremely weak logic in this analogical argument. Correct form but the basic similarity (that people weren't advised) doesn't count in any way towards the propriety of not advising them. (This raises concerns about charity in paraphrasing the argument—but I can't think of an implicit similarity that would be relevant.) And there is an important relevant dissimilarity. The investigations by the university administration apparently had nothing to do with criminality while Hoover's (presumably) did.

SOUNDNESS
Unsound, due to weak logic.

5.

1. Animals in zoos are not dangerous and executing them would be bad for our sense of humanity.
2. Murderers in jail are not dangerous.
∴ C. Executing murderers in jail would be bad for our sense of humanity.

EVALUATION
TRUTH
Premise 1. This is almost certainly true. My experience is that most humans feel enough empathy with animals in a zoo that they regret having them locked up at all, unless it can be justified

as somehow contributing to a greater good for the animal or the species. So, shooting them would be an outrage.

Premise 2. This is certainly true—jail generally protects the rest of us from them.

L<small>OGIC</small>

Extremely weak analogical argument. Correct form, and the similarity has some relevance, since we do feel that killing either an animal or a person who is dangerous (in self-defense) does not significantly diminish our sense of humanity. But the dissimilarity is compelling. The animals are not behind bars for profound wrongdoing, while murderers are.

S<small>OUNDNESS</small>

Unsound, due to weak logic.

7.

1. A child or a $32 million Van Gogh painting is irreplaceable, and danger to it would justify illegally demolishing a tractor.
2. A 400-year-old original growth tree is irreplaceable, though not as irreplaceable as a child or a $32 million Van Gogh painting
∴ C. Danger to a 400-year-old original growth tree would justify illegally demolishing a tractor.

EVALUATION

T<small>RUTH</small>

Premise 1. Probably true—certainly true in the case of the child, less certain in the case of the Van Gogh, but still probable (as long as the driver is not endangered), since a tractor can be replaced.

Premise 2. It is important to be careful here about slippage in the meaning of the term "irreplaceable." If it means "as irreplaceable as a $32 million Van Gogh," then it is clearly false. There are a lot of 400-year-old original growth trees and precious few Van Goghs. And the trees can be replaced in the long run (in 400 years), while Van Gogh will never paint again. But, since I have paraphrased it using the reasonable-premises strategy, the premise is probably true—for practical purposes it is irreplaceable, but not to the same extent as a Van Gogh.

LOGIC
No logical support. In order to make the second premise true, the argument has been clarified so that the basic property turns out not to be the same in each case. So, the argument doesn't have correct form for an argument from analogy.

SOUNDNESS
The argument is unsound, since it is illogical.

9. I leave this one for classroom discussion.

CHAPTER 16, SET (A)
1.   Fallacy of affirming the consequent
   1. If the roof is leaking, then the house needs work.
   2. The house needs work.
∴   C. The roof is leaking.

Explanatory argument
   3. If the roof is leaking, then there will be a stain on the ceiling.
   4. There is a stain on the ceiling.
∴   C. The roof is leaking.

3.   Fallacy of affirming the consequent
   1. If my watch stops, then I own something that isn't functioning properly.
   2. I own something that isn't functioning properly.
∴   C. My watch stopped.

Explanatory argument
   1. If my watch stops, then the hands don't move.
   2. The hands don't move.
∴   C. My watch stopped.

CHAPTER 16, SET (B)

1.

> [1. If somebody mishandled the frame, then there would be a
> tiny dent in the frame.]
>   2. There was a tiny dent in the frame.

∴   C. Somebody mishandled the frame.

Singular explanation. Observable outcome came first.

3.

> [1. If it was an earthquake, then I would hear a funny roar and
> the plants would start to shake without any breeze.]
>   2. I heard a funny roar and the plants started to shake without
> any breeze.

∴   C. It was an earthquake.

Singular explanation. Observable outcome came first.

5.

> [1. If UV radiation is harmful to amphibian populations, then a
> significantly larger number of frog eggs would hatch when UV
> radiation is filtered out than when it is not.]
>   2. A significantly larger number of frog eggs hatched when UV
> radiation was filtered out than when it was not.

∴   C. UV radiation is harmful to amphibian populations

General explanation. Explanation comes first. (It doesn't come
before the declining populations were noted—but that isn't the
observable outcome; the outcome is the big difference between
the results with the shielded and unshielded eggs.)

CHAPTER 16, SET (C)

1. It is the broader explanation—that there is such a thing as
parapsychology (see the phrase "is actually evidence in favor of
parapsychology") that is rendered unfalsifiable by the proviso that
skepticism wipes out the results of successful experiments when the
skeptic reads about them afterwards. The observable outcome of
parapsychology's truth would be that either there *is* evidence for it
(which would simply falsify the proviso, not parapsychology itself) or
that there is *no* evidence for it (which the proviso entails). The
observable outcome that there is or isn't evidence for it, then, is

certain (and so has an extremely high prior probability) and thus the first part of the total evidence condition is not satisfied.

CHAPTER 16, SET (D)

1. Explanation: My car is running low on gas. Observable outcome: My car will run out of gas within the next 10 miles.
3. Explanation: Smoking causes cancer. Observable outcome: Everybody who smokes immediately gets cancer, and nobody else does.
5. Explanation: My employer values me. Observable outcome: My salary will be at least doubled by the first of next month.

CHAPTER 16, SET (E)

1. Alternative explanation: The age and bad condition of the house mean that the electrical wiring is faulty.
3. Alternative explanation: Human nature is such that human beings from different cultures and with radically different goals and needs can be expected to have trouble coming to an understanding.

CHAPTER 16, SET (F)

1. Observable outcome: I lost weight when I regularly lunched at the Thai restaurant. Improved outcome: I lost weight when I regularly lunched at the Thai restaurant and got no additional exercise.
3. Observable outcome: Our friends soon got pregnant. Improved outcome. Our friends soon got pregnant without any sort of fertility intervention. (Note that it isn't clear whether there has been fertility intervention, but the argument is stronger if it is explicitly ruled out.)
5. Observable outcome: There were no asthma attacks after Carter stopped taking asthma medications. Improved outcome: There were no asthma attacks after Carter stopped taking asthma medications and without any other sort of therapeutic intervention.

CHAPTER 16, SET (G)

1. Explanation: The dog ate the student's homework. It is the sort of thing that is known to happen. (I was amazed to learn this when I had a puppy a few years ago!) But students fail to do homework far more frequently than dogs eat it.
3. Explanation: Aliens from outer space visited and did something funny with the trees. It is *not* the sort of thing that is known to

happen—though it is claimed by some to be true, it is, at best, highly controversial. Beavers, however, do frequently take down trees for dams in exactly the way described.

5. Explanation: There is a problem with the young man's phone line that does not affect the dial tone. This is the sort of thing that is known to happen, though it is extremely rare. Far more common is the experience of someone failing to place a call to begin with.

7. Explanation: The suspect was using gas to start his car and poured some near the burning building because the jug was too full. It is, I presume, something that is known to happen. But it is very rare that: (a) someone who is out of gas would waste any on the ground when it is all needed in the car; (b) someone would carelessly pour out gas near a fire (and the frequency of both together is even lower). Molotov cocktails are also rare, but more frequent than the explanation offered.

CHAPTER 16, SET (H)

1. Explanation: Icebergs capsize and expose yellowish-brown organic material from frozen sea water on their underside. This account makes good sense—it fits in with the way we understand the world to work. The only alternative explanations I can think of—emeralds in the icebergs, aliens from outer space painting them green, etc., don't fit into our conceptual framework, i.e., don't make any sense at all.

3. Explanation: There is a planet orbiting pulsar star PSR1829. The explanation makes sense in terms of gravitational effects of an orbiting body. The alternative—that there is some strange effect inside the pulsar—isn't filled out enough yet to make sense; it is, in effect, a way of saying that the alternative is that we don't know the explanation.

CHAPTER 16, SET (I)

1.

[1. If a prehistoric culture sculpted the topographical likeness of George Bernard Shaw on the southern tip of an island in Quebec, then the southern tip of the island in Quebec would resemble George Bernard Shaw.]

2. The southern tip of the island in Quebec resembles George Bernard Shaw.

∴ C. A prehistoric culture sculpted the topographical likeness of

George Bernard Shaw on the southern tip of an island in Quebec.

EVALUATION

TRUTH

Premise 1 is only somewhat probably true. One secondary assumption is simply that a sculpted likeness usually resembles the thing of which it is intended to be a likeness—even in prehistoric times. This is consistent with my experience—more often than not those who are doing the sculpting have some ability at getting it right. Another closely related assumption is that topographical sculptures succeed as often as do other likenesses. This seems less likely—to carve out a successful likeness on a coastline would be pretty hard.

Premise 2 is certainly true—I base this on having seen a photograph of it.

LOGIC

Extremely weak explanatory argument. The form is correct, and the argument does succeed on the first part of the total evidence condition: for any topographical feature, the prior probability that it would resemble George Bernard Shaw is extremely low. But it does poorly on the second part of the total evidence condition: it makes no sense at all. We have no conceptual framework for how a prehistoric culture would know what he looks like centuries before Shaw's existence, why they would want to reproduce his face in this way, and how they would pull it off.

SOUNDNESS

Unsound argument, due to weak logic.

3.

[1. If the police officers in the San Jose State study were suffering from sleep deprivation, then the police officers in the San Jose State study would have given tickets to significantly more of the drivers they stopped at night than in the daytime.]

2. The police officers in the San Jose State study gave tickets to significantly more of the drivers they stopped at night than in the daytime.

∴ C. The police officers in the San Jose State study were suffering from sleep deprivation.

EVALUATION
TRUTH
Premise 1 has as a secondary assumption that a testy police officer is likely to impose a more severe sanction than one who isn't testy. This is almost certainly true. But another assumption is that sleep deprivation tends to make people testy. Probably—but I'm not sure—since in my experience it can also make people inattentive and careless, which might make an officer *less* likely to impose more severe sanctions. Probably it produces more testiness than carelessness, so I'd say the premise is somewhat probably true.
Premise 2 is probably true—I have no reason to doubt the news report or the psychologists.

LOGIC
Extremely weak explanatory argument. Correct form, but the argument does poorly on the first part of the total evidence condition. The observable outcome has a fairly high prior probability; it wouldn't be surprising even if they weren't sleep deprived, since in my experience those who do exceed the speed limit at night exceed it by greater amounts (since there is less traffic)—thus, they are objectively more worthy of tickets. Neither does it do well on the first part of the total evidence condition. This explanation, of course, has a reasonably high prior probability; people up late at night do tend to suffer from sleep deprivation. But the argument has not ruled out another alternative; perhaps the same set of officers always works the night shift (and thus, being used to it, suffers very little from sleep deprivation) and, by chance, they happen to be officers who are more ticket-happy. This needs to be ruled out.

SOUNDNESS
Unsound, due to weak logic.

5.

      [1. If TM can affect the weather, then when materials were
      available and MIU students were instructed to desire warm
      weather, there would be warm weather on the next day.]

    2. When materials were available and MIU students were
       instructed to desire warm weather there was warm weather on
       the next day.

∴   C. TM can affect the weather.

EVALUATION

TRUTH

Premise 1 is probably true. A secondary assumption is that the
MIU students did what they were told, and that they knew the
proper techniques. This is probably true.

Premise 2 is probably true. There is no reason to doubt the
reliability of Rabinoff, Trumpy, or the *Skeptical Inquirer* on
this count.

LOGIC

Extremely weak explanatory argument. Form is correct, but the
observable outcome turns out to have a high prior probability.
Even if TM cannot effect weather, we would expect warm
weather when the materials were available since the materials
were prepared only when warm weather was forecast. The
second part of the total evidence condition is also problematic—
nobody yet has any account of how TM might have this sort of
effect—there is no conceptual framework for understanding it,
nor any clear reason to believe it has ever happened before.

SOUNDNESS

Unsound, due to logical weakness.

NOTES

NOTES

112

NOTES

113

NOTES

NOTES

NOTES